Table of Contents

Introduction

I must admit that I was pleasantly thrilled with the reception of the first Table Lessons: Insights in the Practice of Massage Therapy book. So many therapists contacted me to say that the book resonated with them, especially the clinical stories that involved struggle and seeming failure. I think all of us feel alone and on the front lines at some point, doing our best for the clients we see but wondering if we are missing something or up to the task when things don't go well.

In the end, it is the clients with whom we struggle that provide us with the greatest opportunity for learning and growth. Being pushed to explore new ground is part of the clinical experience. As the saying goes, "If it doesn't challenge you, it doesn't change you." In reality, every client contact is an opportunity for learning and a deeper understanding. Sometimes it is a technical understanding, sometimes a lesson in "people-ology". In any case, each connection has the potential to make us better therapists and better people as well. Like so many other aspects of life, these windows of opportunity don't open by themselves, we must recognize and seize them and the breath of fresh air they can provide.

It is my sincere wish that you find pearls of wisdom in these stories that you can apply to your practice. Moreover, I hope they inspire you to explore the Table Lessons waiting to unfold each day in your clinic or office.

Douglas Nelson

Chapter One: Challenges

*"We know that how you think affects
how you feel. There is very strong
evidence to the reverse as well;
how you feel affects how you think."*

Placated[NK1]?

I have had the great fortune to work with many excellent Certified Athletic Trainers (ATC's) during my years of working with collegiate and professional athletes. Over time, these trainers know when to refer to me and which conditions respond favorably to soft-tissue therapy. Many have been excellent at assessment, which is often the hardest part of treatment. In my regular office, I need to spend time figuring out the cause of my client's pain. When working with these excellent ATC's in the sports environment, they have already done that for me; I just need to do the work. What a luxury that is! This long history of working with great ATC's is why my experience with a new trainer was so startling. I had been seeing one player after the other but had a bit of a break while waiting for another athlete to make it from the training room to my treatment area. During that break, the new ATC popped in to introduce himself and see how things were going.

"Everything going well?" he asked. "The players really seem to like a massage; which is probably a very good thing. Sometimes, athletes just need to be placated."

I was stunned at his statement. Absolutely gob-smacked. "Placated? You are kidding me. Is that what he thinks I am doing?" I thought to myself. I was too floored to respond at that moment, but I knew I couldn't let the comment pass without addressing it. That chance came after I finished treating the last athlete. Gathering up my things, I happened to run into this trainer on my way out of the building. (Okay, perhaps I did take a circuitous route hoping I would run into him.)

"If you have a second, I'd like to share with you the methodology behind what I am doing with the players. I know that what I am doing looks rather simple, but the thought process is quite deep and connected to your focus on muscular function. I don't use tools or machines, just my hands. The complexity isn't in what you see, but in what you cannot.

May I give you an example? Let's imagine that an athlete has pain in the anterior shoulder, for instance," I posited.

"Like my left shoulder?" the trainer asked with interest.

Wow. Only so many times do you get such a perfect example handed to you. I was not going to miss this opportunity.

"Really," I replied. "I'm curious. If I strength test your left anterior deltoid relative to your right shoulder, is the left deltoid weaker?"

"You can test it if you want, but I can tell you right now it is significantly weaker than the right deltoid. I have been doing strengthening exercises, but it doesn't get stronger and the pain seems to increase after exercise. I have been working on that issue for almost three months."

The massage gods were clearly smiling on me.

Just to double-check (and to emphasize the point), I did perform the resistive testing on the left anterior deltoid and found it significantly weaker than his right. Resistive testing of the left deltoid also created some discomfort during the contraction as well.

"Are you familiar with trigger points?" I asked the trainer.

"Sure," he said. "They are specific points that refer pain to other parts of the body."

"That's true, but only part of the story," I answered. "It is more accurate to say that trigger points refer sensation, rather than pain. Sometimes trigger points mimic nerve entrapment, a feeling of itching, or perhaps even nausea. More commonly, trigger points can create motor inhibition in areas of referral, making muscles in the area of referral test weak. This phenomenon is called motor inhibition and is much more common than most therapists realize. This presentation of weakness may be even more common than the existence of pain.

As an example, the common referral area for the infraspinatus happens to be the anterior deltoid. It is possible that an infraspinatus trigger point can create a deep ache in the anterior deltoid, but another possibility is that the infraspinatus can create motor inhibition of the anterior deltoid, decreasing its strength. Let me show you."

Using my thumb to examine his infraspinatus, I happened to land on exactly the right spot. (Sometimes, it is better to be lucky than good.) Pressing on the tiny nodule I felt in his left infraspinatus, he felt an immediate deep aching in the front of his left shoulder. Judging by his reaction, the spot was exquisitely tender.

"Holy crap (he might have used another work with the same meaning), that is crazy," he exclaimed. "It feels like you are digging into the anterior deltoid and you aren't even touching it. That's wild. If I had my eyes closed, I'd swear you were pressing in the front of my shoulder. Man, oh man, is that tender!"

I probably should have let it go, but I couldn't resist responding to his earlier comment. Keeping the pressure on the point in his infraspinatus, I asked another question.

"Just curious, how placated do you feel right now?"

(The massage gods were now jumping out of their seats and cheering.)

The knowing look on his face said it all as I released pressure on the trigger point. He just looked perplexed, curious, and more than a little embarrassed.

"Welcome to the mysterious world of trigger points and referred sensation. Wild, isn't it? Now, let's check something. Hold out your left arm and let's strength test the anterior deltoid again," I instructed.

This time, his left deltoid was significantly stronger, testing approximately the same strength as his right side. The incredulous look on his face said it all. What weeks of targeted strengthening exercises could not accomplish was changed in less than one minute.

"That is amazing," he said. "I would have never believed it, but the strength difference is astounding."

"That is what I am doing with the players," I said. "It may not be exciting to watch, but there is a complicated methodology behind these treatments. My job is to address areas of restriction and motor inhibited weakness, both of which may decrease performance and be the product of trigger point referral. Ultimately, my job is to maximize the effectiveness of your work with players, making targeting exercise more effective. With your left shoulder, you should see a progressive strength increase over the next week or two. Now is the time to load it gradually, so that you can keep the progress we just made. Together, we are a powerful team. The effect of what I just did would fade over time if you did not challenge the deltoid and put the newfound strength to use. However, strength training alone won't improve this problem without addressing the tissue. You know; you already tried that to no avail. We have to work together."

He nodded in approval. "I still find it amazing that a tiny spot in one muscle can make another muscle weak," he mused.

"So do I," I concurred. "After all these years, it still blows me away how much difference something so small can make."

Addendum

Just for the record, this ATC went on to become one of the biggest cheerleaders for my work I have ever had. The last I heard, he was now in medical school studying musculoskeletal medicine. Wherever he is, you can bet he is referring patients to massage therapy. His respect for this field is deep and wide.

One never knows the impact you have on people. Our little connection was pivotal to his career. His future patients will be the beneficiaries of that connection.

Confident Enough to Fail

I met J's father unexpectedly at a social event. A no-nonsense executive, he called me aside to ask if I might look at his daughter's shoulder pain, an issue that she had been struggling with for too long. I met with them both the next evening, adding her to my (already very long) day.

"It first began as a pain in my shoulder, somewhere around here," stated J, pointing to her right upper trapezius area. "I thought it would go away, but it just kept hanging on, getting slowly worse. That's when we went to see the doctor. "

"The doctor sent us to physical therapy," added her dad. "They diagnosed it as scapular instability. She has been going for therapy two to three times a week for almost four months. She is getting stronger, but the pain is really about the same as it was in the beginning. J is a two-sport athlete and a very good one. I don't want this condition to affect her playing soccer or volleyball."

J nodded, showing frustration on her face at the thought of not being able to play the sports that she loves so much.

"Okay, I understand how this pain affects your participation in sports," I stated. "But is that when you feel it the most?"

"Yes, at first it only hurt when I was playing. Over time, it kept hurting even when I wasn't playing. Even now though, it is far worse when I play. I have to severely limit my playing time if I can play at all."

"Is there a certain movement or action that makes it hurt the most?" I inquired.

"Yes. Running," answered J emphatically.

"Running," I restated, looking at both of them while I was lost in thought.

What followed was one of those moments where, like Alice, I was lost down the rabbit hole of a cascade of thoughts. Shoulder instability? I understand that this is a common diagnosis for athletes, especially young females, but this makes absolutely no sense if her pain is worse when she runs. Moreover, if four months of multiple treatments per week haven't helped, it is kind of a clue that instability isn't the problem. This was hardly effective or efficient therapy. Coming back to the moment at hand, I decided to take a different course.

"Could you lie on the table on your left side for me? I want to check something that perhaps no one else has treated. Actually, has anyone actually used their hands to explore the soft tissue of your shoulder?"

"No, I guess not," replied J, getting on the table.

The first thought I had that would explain her symptoms was the serratus posterior superior. It often presents as a deep scapular ache, which often refers down the arm. An ancillary respiratory muscle, it would be used in high volume breathing. I slowly moved J's scapula anteriorly to reveal the distal attachments of the serratus.

"Wow, that's tender," she exclaimed. "I can feel that sensation spreading throughout my shoulder."

Glancing at her father, I could see him widening his eyes, trying to understand what I was doing. I explained to him what this muscle was and why it is a reasonable fit for J's pain.

"You mean that we have done months of therapy, but the source of her pain could have been this muscle the whole time?"

Some questions are best left unanswered. I just looked at him. "Theories are easy, results are hard. If I'm right, we will see results. If not, that will also be clear. Contact me in four days after she has vigorously exercised. Let's see if this makes a difference. The proof is in the pudding."

Four days and two soccer practices later, there was no appreciable improvement. With their approval, I scheduled session number two.

"I'm curious to see how that muscle is doing," stated J's father.

"I'm not even going to check it," I replied. "Same game, new strategy."

"Really," questioned J's dad. "So soon? It just seems kind of fast. I thought the muscle you treated last time would be the answer. Now you don't seem so sure," he responded. There was something in his tone that alluded to a lack of confidence or indecisiveness on my part.

"When I don't get the results I want, I switch strategies. Confidence is also the willingness and openness to change course when the results don't justify the approach. If we were on the right course, we'd have results. I think we should expand the search," I asserted.

"Confidence doesn't make you correct, results do. If I might add, how confident were the therapists that the source of your daughter's pain was scapular instability?" I challenged.

"Very," he replied sheepishly. He was a little quiet from this point, thinking about the broader implications.

As I returned to thinking about what might be involved in respiration and running, it occurred to me that I should have checked the posterior scalene. Asking J if she happened to notice anything else that made the pain worse, she said holding her arms up in the air in volleyball was a trigger. Since the levator scapula is stretched in upward rotation of the scapula, I added treatment of that muscle too.

Days later, I got a text from her father, who was thrilled with her results. J played four soccer games and two volleyball practices without pain. I have seen them both several times since then, and for different athletic injuries. Just so you know, J's dad has never questioned the approach.

Quackery? Seriously?

During advanced training at my office, people who have select soft tissue problems are invited to receive treatment from myself with a small number of my advanced students present. V was one of those lucky few on our schedule; I turn away about ten people for every client we can accept. Knowing how competitive it is for one of these appointments, I was a little surprised at V's distant attitude.

"Tell me again how you were referred to me?" I asked.

"Essentially, my wife encouraged me to come. This isn't something I would typically do, as I teach at the university," he replied.

I thought to myself what a strange comment that was, but also surmised that perhaps I may not have heard him correctly. I let it go.

"I have had knee pain for many years, probably dating back to when I was playing football in college. My left knee is much worse than the right. I had arthroscopic surgery for arthritic changes in my left knee about two years ago, but it did not help. Lately, I have been diagnosed with patellofemoral syndrome, but the treatment for that condition hasn't really helped me either. My knee pain is seriously affecting my daily life."

"Is there some action you can do that consistently initiates the pain?" I inquired.

"That's easy. It hurts every single time I bend it," V answered.

Sure enough, the pain on his face was obvious after bending his knee about thirty degrees. V stated that his pain was only during weight-bearing and that passive motion of the knee was not typically painful. The pain was generally at the medial knee, but the distribution of the discomfort seemed fairly broad.

Having just reviewed several tests for patellofemoral syndrome with my students, we went right to work. It was at this point that the assessment train began to derail! None of the standard tests for patellar tracking issues showed positive, in direct conflict with his diagnosis. That left me in an uncomfortable position, especially in front of my students. There were two possible explanations- either the tests did not pick up his condition (then why should we use them?) or V does not have patellofemoral syndrome. This was a conundrum; I certainly did not want to question or conflict with his diagnosis in front of him or my students. Yet, the tests did not point that direction. What to do. . .

I decided to act quickly, choosing to treat V as if he had patellofemoral syndrome anyway. Examining carefully his vastus lateralis, I was surprised to find nothing remarkable in it or the iliotibial band. I carefully examined his vastus medialis, thinking that perhaps a trigger point had created motor inhibition, but no trigger points were found. Asking him to stand again, V tried a small squat.

"Still there," he said. "No change."

"Well, that was remarkably unsuccessful!" I said, stating the obvious. "Lie down again and let's try a different approach."

What followed was a series of multiple strategies that might account for his pain. I would treat several muscles and then have him stand up and retest. Each time, his pain was unchanged. On the fifth approach, targeting the popliteus muscle, V stood up again, and I could tell he was losing patience. Squatting, his face brightened, then a return to straight legs, then another squat.

"Oh my goodness," he exclaimed. "I can't believe it! This is great; I can squat with no pain!"

I couldn't resist teasing him a bit. "I'd appreciate it if you didn't act so surprised. We are supposed to get results. That's the point!" I stated, thinking I was clever.

"I can't help it," he said. "I'm really surprised. I didn't think this therapy would help. I, umm, teach at the university."

There was that comment again, and this time I had to ask.

"What does teaching at the university have to do with this?" I inquired.

"Well," he said, "I teach a class on community health and one of the modules is on quackery." (I still looked confused as he was saying this.) "Massage therapy is in that module."

It took a moment for that last statement to sink in.

"Quackery? Seriously? You teach a section on quackery and massage therapy is in there?"

V looked a little sheepish, which was perfectly appropriate given the present pain-free state of his knee. He should have been embarrassed.

"How old is the text you are using? Actually, never mind," I stated. "I have a better idea. If you'd like, I'd be happy to speak to your class about the science behind massage therapy."

V happily agreed to have me speak to his class and he left my office with a big grin and a bounce in his step not present when he arrived an hour earlier.

About every six weeks or so, I continued to check on V's status, and in each email, he informed me that his knee has been fine. While I was thrilled with the treatment results, I was a bit discouraged, as none of these emails contained an invitation to speak to his class.

That invitation came finally came about four months after his initial visit. I spoke to his class of about two hundred students on a Monday morning. I found it interesting on several levels, one being that there were several clients in my office in his class and they were huge fans. Since these clients happened to be very well-known student-athletes, it did get the students' attention when they were psyched about the value of massage therapy. Speaking to the class about the research underpinnings of massage and the work of the Massage Therapy Foundation, I think these young people left the class with a very different view of the field than whatever his old text would have given them. He and his class needed better information. It's up to us to make it available. (That is also why I am passionate about the research efforts of the Massage Therapy Foundation.)

Chapter Two: Reprogramming

"Simple and easy are not the same thing.
As a mentor of mine pointed out, telling
the truth is simple but seldom easy."

A New Normal

My client T entered my treatment room wearing a smile from ear to ear while saying, "My back hasn't felt this good in a long time."

These are the kind of statements one loves to hear to begin a session.

"Any spasms since our last session?" I inquired, wondering what direction the session would take us.

"Not since before my last visit, even with the longer time span in between appointments. To be honest, I felt good enough that I considered canceling but decided to come in anyway. I felt such a difference after both of the sessions, but the effect wore off after about three days," T stated.

"In the last session we focused on the muscles of your back, but we need to spend some time with your hips today," I said, laying out the game plan. "The more restricted your hips are, the more your low back tries to compensate by moving more. That can be problematic for the back, which seeks stability, not excessive mobility. Keeping your hips as mobile as possible will be preventive for your back. It's easier to prevent a problem than to solve a problem."

I asked T to lie prone on the table while I gently assessed femoral internal and external rotation. Finding his internal rotation quite restricted, I targeted the quadratus femoris and the piriformis, looking for tight and tender areas.

Suddenly, I could hear muffled laughter through the face rest.

"Are you okay?" I asked.

"I don't understand how you seem to know right where the problem is, but maybe more importantly, how can I be so unaware of something that hurts so much? Wouldn't you think I would know about muscles that are that painful?"

"That is a fabulous question and one I hear from a lot of people. In a way, it is similar to what you mentioned earlier about having the beneficial effect of a session wear off in two or three days."

"How are they related? They seem opposite," T asked.

"The principle revolves around the concept of what you perceive as normal. How does your brain decide what to pay attention to and what to ignore? As it turns out, this is an important question and one that the brain assigns a lot of bandwidth trying to solve. Much of the physical sense of "normal" happens in an area of the brain called the cerebellum. While the cerebellum is just 10% of brain volume, it contains about 50% of the neurons of the brain. A big part of its job is discerning the expected from the unexpected. For instance, soon after putting on a shirt in the morning, you no longer notice the shirt sleeve rubbing against your arm while you move. Why not? In the myriad of sensations that the brain has the capability to sense, it has to prioritize."

"That makes sense, but where you were pressing is really painful. You'd think that kind of pain would have gotten my attention earlier. Why wouldn't I notice it?" asked T.

"The brain generally asks three questions of every new sensation: What is it? What does it mean? What do I do? It is highly likely that at one time, you were aware of some discomfort or restriction in your hips. As time went on, however, the sensation of restriction didn't change significantly in either direction, signaling to your brain that this discomfort is not a severe threat and can be ignored until further review. It became your new normal. It is important to realize that the new normal doesn't feel any different than the old normal. In fact, time dulls memory of the old normal. Only when you can contrast them within a tight timeframe is there any possibility of a true comparison," I explained.

"You said that is connected to my improvements after the earlier sessions. How so?" asked T.

"After our first two sessions, your body experienced a remarkable difference. Since this change happened so fast, you could really compare and contrast the changes immediately, making the difference abundantly clear. The increase in painless movement was dramatic, but the novelty of that change fades over time as the increased range becomes the new normal. Most people only notice these differences when they notice a change in the ease of movement when doing a familiar daily activity. That activity could be getting in and out of a car, reaching into the top shelf for a coffee cup, or picking up a child; something they do all the time and have a way to notice the ease with which they move.

"Once the improvement is sustained, the novelty of that wears off as well. You are in good company; many other people have also stated that the benefits they initially noticed faded after three days. It is only when I point out the increase in their activity level that they realize how much they have improved."

"It seems like the perception of normal can work in both directions; it explains how we get worse without noticing, or how incremental improvements can be overlooked as well. What we call normal is a constantly moving target," surmised T.

"That is exactly correct," I responded. "Our perception of self depends on consistent, accurate, and timely information about the state of our body, and massage is excellent at revealing the nervous system to itself."

"Well, the message I am getting from the body is that my hips are way too tight," T commented, with a mischievous smile.

"Message received. Let's see what we can do about that," I replied, exploring the muscular anatomy of his hip with renewed focus.

A Software Problem

"Thanks for checking in with me," I said, taking a call from a client I had seen three weeks earlier. "I hope you are a bit better, especially since you drove so far for the appointment."

"Not just a bit better, a lot better," she said. "The pain is almost completely gone. I am thrilled."

Given that Mrs. G had suffered from nearly constant pain in her left buttock, this was great news.

With any presenting problem, the old adage applies- One Symptom; Many Possible Causes. Mrs. G's pain could have been due to a multitude of factors: the piriformis, hip joint pathology, sacroiliac joint dysfunction (SIJ), trigger point referral, or a spinal facet issue. The task of the therapist is to go through a list of possible reasons, looking for information that will confirm or rule out each of these possibilities.

My first question was whether the pain was worse in sitting, standing, or walking.

"Sitting is fine, but I cannot stand or walk for very long," she responded.

This is a simple but very important question. Pain during walking and relieved while sitting could implicate arthritic changes in the hip. However, standing does not typically bother an arthritic hip.

I asked Mrs. G to lie supine on the massage table while I checked her left internal femoral rotation, which was even greater on the involved left hip than the right. External rotation of her left femur against resistance also elicited no pain. With full range (external rotation and flexion were also normal) and non-painful contraction, neither hip pathology or piriformis issues seemed likely. This could be removed from the list, or at least moved down to be addressed later if we were unsuccessful. Testing isn't perfect, it is more about probability than something definitive.

Deciding to move from testing to palpation, careful examination of the iliocostalis and the costal attachments of the quadratus lumborum revealed very sensitive areas, but none of which referred to the buttock. If the source of the pain is a referral, then I should be able to recreate the symptoms using palpation. Since I could not, a trigger point referral was also taken off the list. Next up!

To explore facet compression, I rotated her lumbar spine to the right (which did not recreate her pain), but left rotation caused an immediate reaction.

"Oh my gosh, that feels great," she said. "I feel a wave of relief from my spine to my hips." Score one for facet compression. I then asked her to lie on the massage table on her right side. I put a small pillow under her right lumbar spine to create slight decompression on the left lumbar spine. Grasping her left hip, I pulled it slightly forward while also rotating her spine to the left. This position decompresses the left lumbar facets. She felt waves of relief as I did so. I continued to hold Mrs. G in that spinal position as long as it felt relieving to her. We would come into and out of it slowly, doing this repeatedly. I felt that the facet issue was important, but not the whole story.

To address the possibility of a problem with the Sacroiliac joint (SIJ), I did several tests, none of which were positive. Reflecting on the decompressive relief she had from the spine, I tried the same strategy with her SIJ. With her lying in the supine position and knees bent, I put one hand under her sacrum, pressing it anterior in relation to both innominates. She immediately experienced a wave of relaxation throughout the involved area.

Decompression of both the facet and the SIJ provided immediate relief. But why didn't compression elicit symptoms? Why wasn't the reverse also true? If decompression creates relief, compression should elicit symptoms. Perplexed, I asked her to stand and point to the epicenter of pain. Guided by her hand, I felt obvious soft tissue restriction. Just as I was about to say something, the muscle under my finger relaxed.

"Are you in pain now? I asked. "No, it just stopped," she responded. Suddenly, the muscle under my finger contracted again and she immediately reported that the pain had returned.

"Feel this with me," I requested, as I guided her hand to the spot in question. As she did, the muscle alternately relaxed (relieving the pain) and contracted (causing the pain to return.)

"Let's try using your hand as a feedback system to monitor muscular activity. Try to make the muscle contract and then relax it. Figure out how to do that."

"I don't know how to do that," she admitted. "How do I make that happen?"

"How would I know?" I teased. She gave me a look of surprise. "Actually, I'm not kidding. I'm not sure what to tell you. In fact, anything I tell you will probably get in the way. You just need to figure it out for yourself. You have a great feedback through your hands. Figure out what works. No one can tell you what to do."

As she was experimenting, I was lost in thought about some research I read a few years ago. With new technology, it is possible to see brain activity. The brain region being studied in this particular study was the insula. An increase in insular activity is vital for interoception - one's awareness of self.

In the study, the researchers put the subject in a small room with a monitor. The screen showed insular activity. The goal was to change the color (and therefore the activity of the insula) from red to green. The obvious question from the subjects was something to the effect of, "And how the heck do I do that?"

Essentially, the researchers would smile and then leave the room (those dastardly grad students!). Subjects would breathe like they think they are supposed to, the color got even redder. Imagining themselves on an island, again, redder. Finally giving up, giving in, and foregoing all the stuff that people told them was relaxing, they just figured it out on their own. What works for one does not apply to all. Find your own way.

After many failures and intermittent successes, Mrs. G was able to contract and relax the muscle selectively. As expected, she would succeed and then fail again. As time passed, (it probably seemed like an eternity for her), she was able to relax the muscle consistently.

"That is crazy," she said in amazement. "I never realized I could control my muscles like that."

"Your pain is likely to be more of a software problem than a hardware problem. For whatever reason, this muscle was firing randomly and inappropriately. Learning to selectively contract and relax the muscle can help rewrite the program, like rewriting the software on a computer," I shared with her.

At the end of the session, I reviewed with her the three possible sources of her pain: facet decompression, SIJ, and muscle reprogramming. Each had a self-care component: spinal twist for facet decompression, a rolled towel in place of my hand to decompress the SIJ and do the muscle reprogramming daily.

Returning to our current phone conversation, I wanted to know which of the three strategies was most helpful, thus revealing the ultimate source of her pain.

"I don't know," she said. "Perhaps the most helpful aspect of the session was that I felt empowered to know there were things I could do to help myself. If I felt the pain, I practiced contracting and relaxing. If that did not work, I did the spinal twist or the towel under the sacrum. I don't know if one of the three was primary; I am just thrilled the pain is essentially gone."

In a perfect world, the source of Mrs. G's pain would be clearly reduced to a singular cause. In the slightly messier world in which we practice, symptoms often result from the convergence of multiple factors. We need to deal with them in a multifaceted approach to be successful, and, if possible, find ways to involve the client in the process as well.

[NK2]Always On

"First, I want to tell you that my leg has been better ever since you treated it last month. I haven't given it a thought for weeks. That's not the pressing issue for today," Mrs. M said, taking off her coat. "I have a new issue; this muscle right here," she stated, as she pointed to her upper trapezius muscle. "I can't shut it off. It's like there is a switch somewhere that is stuck in the 'on' position and I can't find the switch."

"What a great metaphor," I remarked. "There has to be a switch somewhere. Let's see if we can find it!"

I had Mrs. M lie supine on my massage table as I began to examine her right upper trapezius with very slow and careful pressure using flat palpation. Almost immediately, Mrs. M declared the tissue I first landed on to be tender and likely the source of her tension. After a bit, the sensitivity began to subside. Moving just a few centimeters distally, I immediately happened on another spot that Mrs. M declared to be important. After that spot also released, I again moved just slightly, only to discover another "important" area. At this point, my alarm bell went off. That is too many areas of seeming importance. I decided to confirm that idea.

"I'd like to explore the whole area a bit more quickly if you don't mind," I told Mrs. M. Doing so, almost everything I touched was quite tender, each one about the same as the last.

"I don't like this, I told her. "It seems there are too many sensitive points in your shoulder. My experience in the past is that, if everything is it, nothing is it. It's like playing whack-a-mole with pain. I'd like to try something. Could you lie on your left side?"

With Mrs. M on her left side, I sat behind her and wrapped my right hand around the front of her shoulder while placing my left hand over her scapula. I began to slowly move her whole shoulder into elevation, depression, protraction, and retraction. The point of this movement was to sense resistance, assessing which movements were easy and which movements were difficult. Moving her shoulder into depression was smooth and effortless, while elevation was rather difficult and, for lack of a better word, ratcheting[NK3].

"Can you feel what I am doing with your shoulder? I asked. "What do you notice?"

"Nothing hurts when you do that if that's what you are asking," she responded.

"I didn't expect it to be painful, but I am curious as to what you perceive about the quality of the movement. Does each direction feel the same? Do they all have the same ease?"

Doing the movements with her shoulder again, Mrs. M paid closer attention. "It seems that when you push my shoulder upwards, I have a hard time just letting you do that. I can feel myself somehow resisting the motion."

"This is what is so interesting," I responded. "If I pull your shoulder downwards towards your feet, which muscles have to let go?"

"The muscles above," Mrs. M replied without hesitation.

"And if I push your shoulder upwards?" I added.

"The muscles from below. Which is curious since where I feel tension is in the muscles from above," she said, pointing to her upper trapezius.

"I have an idea," I asserted. "Let's fully treat the muscles from below and then see what happens."

For the next ten or fifteen minutes, I treated the latissimus dorsi and lower trapezius muscles thoroughly with flat palpation and pincer palpation, finding and treating several sensitive areas. After finishing, I repeated moving her shoulder superiorly and inferiorly. This time, the movement was effortless and easy.

"What a change," Mrs. M observed. "It seems easy now."

"Let's check the upper trapezius muscle again, which is where we started initially," I said, as I had her return to the supine position. Reexamining the previously sensitive areas, there was a substantial improvement. Most of the spots were gone and those left were far less tender. Mrs. M looked a bit perplexed.

"How did treating the muscles below quiet the muscles above?" she inquired.

"Muscles work in opposing pairs during movement. When one pulls upward, it is opposed by another muscle pulling downward. If one muscle contracts, the opposing muscle must turn off," I explained. "These relationships allow us to move with ease and grace. However, when one muscle has unrelenting low-level tension even at rest, it causes the opposing muscle to respond in kind with a low-level contraction of its own. It is a kind of counter-balancing. In your case, the muscles from below keep sending a message that they are contracting, necessitating the other side, your upper trapezius, to counter that contraction with tension of its own. That creates a vicious cycle of tension.”

“So that was my feeling that the muscles were always on?” she asked.

“Exactly, I responded. “When we shut down the tension from below, the tension from above also receded.”

“Muscles are kind of like people in that regard, I suppose; they respond to what they sense around them,” Mrs. M observed.

“Indeed,” I concurred. “Indeed.”

Degenerative Changes: Seeing is Believing

K was an elegant woman in her late seventies. Her many years of dance training were clearly evident in the way she carried herself. When I asked her how I might be of help, her reply was very clear.

"I don't know if you can help, but my friends say you have done wonders for them. My case is probably different from theirs. I have been diagnosed with severe degenerative arthritis of my spine and my right hip. I don't know how much you can do for arthritic degeneration, but I would be happy with any small improvement," K stated, with resignation in her voice.

In reality, K was referred to me by her two friends who cajoled and badgered her into seeing me, as they admitted as much. Both of them confided to me that K was struggling not only with pain but with depression as well. Since they had never known her to be depressed, the reasonable assumption was that the depression was a result of her unrelenting pain. Having K in my office was quite the accomplishment for her friends.

Looking for a way to develop therapeutic alliance with K, I wanted to acknowledge her plight.

"I assume this has been coming on gradually, getting progressively worse," I asserted. "I'm sure that has been very difficult."

"No," she replied, looking at me with the look you give people who are way off the mark. "This started December 20, right before Christmas. It was a stressful time."

"You can name the day?" I inquired, a little stunned.

"Give me some time and I can tell you the exact hour," she stated, rather confidently.

This was not going at all the way I expected. If the problem is degenerative, how could she be so specific?

"What about before December the 20th? How much pain did you have then?"

"Not much, except for being a little stiff in the morning. After the holidays were over and I had more time, I went to see my doctor and he took X-rays. The diagnosis was degenerative arthritis in my lumbar spine and right hip. He said there isn't really anything to do for the back other than taking some medication."

"Show me where your back is hurting," I instructed. K stood and pointed to her low back and sacral area, stating that the pain is bilateral.

While K was standing, I palpated her erector spinae in the lumbar area. Taking her hand, I placed her finger over the muscle. "What do you feel?" I asked.

"I feel my spine," she said.

"Actually, that's a muscle," I replied as she looked at me in disbelief. "It feels hard because it is working like crazy, but this muscle should be fairly relaxed while you are standing." I placed her fingers over the muscle and began altering her position, bringing her over the plane of gravity.

"Oh my goodness, I just felt it soften."

"Exactly," I replied. "By altering your position, the muscle relaxed because the bones in your spine are taking the weight of gravity, not the muscles. Can you feel the difference? Lean forward and feel the muscle contract again. Now, bring your weight back again and feel the muscle relax."

"That's wonderful," she exclaimed, staring at me in amazement. "I can practice this at home too, correct?"

"Exactly," I affirmed. Could you lie on your right side on my table? Let's examine your muscles while you are on the table."

With K lying on her side, I began to palpate her multifidi and erector spinae. While several areas were quite sensitive, it wasn't until I touched the multifidi attachments at about S2 that she reacted strongly.

"Goodness, that is tender," K exclaimed. "No wonder I hurt."

Having K lie on her left side, we went through almost exactly the same procedure with her right multifidi and erector spinae. The areas of tenderness were quite similar bilaterally.

I then turned my attention to her hip, taking it gently through a range of motion in all planes. I was stunned at her movement capability; it was far better than I expected. My face must have looked perplexed.

"Is everything okay?" K inquired.

"Better than okay," I replied. "Your hip has much more movement than I expected, given your diagnosis."

"That's nice to hear, but both doctors said the hip is very arthritic. I am afraid that I won't be able to sustain the active lifestyle that my husband and I have always enjoyed."

"Wait, both doctors?" I asked.

"Yes, a doctor at Mayo Clinic also said that I would likely be using a cane in less than five years. It is quite depressing to have that to look forward to."

"When was that?" I happened to ask.

"1999", she replied nonchalantly. I stared at her in disbelief. It took a moment for her to realize what she just said. That prediction of the demise of her hip was more than fifteen years ago.

K's story revolves around the power of the nocebo effect, and how careful all health care providers must be in response. Placebos create a positive impact, even though they are inert. Nocebos are the exact opposite, creating a negative effect when in reality that should have no effect.

Seeing the X-ray and having a physician point out arthritis can be a powerful emotional experience. In no small part, it was more powerful for K because of the incredibly active lifestyle she and her husband lead (his energy level is legendary, and he is 82!). When K heard the word "degeneration", she imagined her life taking a steep and unrelenting turn for the worse. Gone would be the travel, the active social life, and the exercise classes she loved. What would this mean for her beloved husband? How would her debility affect his life and their relationship? Life would be forever changed.

It was time for a little reason to enter the picture.

"If I may, I'd like to point something out. Since your pain started exactly on December 20, what do you suppose that your spine looked like on December 19th? The word degeneration implies a process, but this started on a particular day, at a particular hour. And by the way, it isn't like "degenerates" move in and take over your spine overnight. None of that makes any sense.

"In addition, it is extremely unusual for anyone over seventy *not* to show degenerative changes in the spine. Almost everyone at your age shows signs of degenerative changes, but only some of them have pain. If degeneration causes pain, then most people with degenerative changes would have pain. They don't.

"To my point, the prediction that you would be using a cane in five years was over fifteen years ago. So much for using the X-ray as a predictor of pain and dysfunction," I asserted, watching carefully for her reaction.

K's facial expression changed slowly as she processed the meaning of my assertion.

"Yeah, wait a minute. That doesn't make any sense. Maybe the X-ray looks worse than it actually is, or that it does not represent how I actually feel," she wondered out loud.

"Absolutely," I agreed. "It is not a given that what is seen on a diagnostic image directly relates to what you feel."

K did indeed improve greatly after two sessions, showing that degenerative changes could not account for all her pain. Obviously, the degenerative changes did not improve, but her pain level was far less, and her activity level was much greater. It is certainly possible, if not likely, that a great deal of her improvement was probably due to a change in her perception of the meaning of her pain. Words and images have powerful effects, both positive (placebo) and negative (nocebo). Images don't always tell the whole story; there isn't always a direct relationship between what is seen and the pain a person is experiencing. Unfortunately, in many cases, seeing is believing.

Quiet the Riot

When S first presented at my office, I knew that this would not be a typical case. I knew that her friends had encouraged her to call me.

"My situation is probably quite different than many of the people you see. To begin with, I am not really in pain; at least, now. I was in a fair amount of pain for quite a few years. The pain was centered right near my left shoulder blade. It was mostly an aching, deep pain that would vary in intensity. It would radiate out to my arm at times, up to my neck at others. When it was in full swing, I could hardly concentrate. It was very uncomfortable. None of the doctors I saw knew what to do, but one of them prescribed a medication which I have been taking now for several years. It has worked very well; as long as I take it, I am not really in any pain.

"Strangely enough, that is why I am here. I am tired of having to take this medication with perhaps no end in sight. If there is a chance to revisit this and perhaps get off the medication, I'd love to try."

"I'd love to explore this with you. Since there were positions and movements that both aggravated it and relieved it, the pain is likely to be soft-tissue related. I think our chances should be quite good at resolving this."

I had S lie on her right side as I began to explore the musculature around her scapula. The first order of business was to determine if this was a scapular issue or a cervical issue. By following the muscle fiber direction, I was able to isolate each muscle I palpated, and I had her move her neck or her scapula to engage the muscle, further clarifying my decisions.

"What do you think it is?" S asked.

"It could be any of four different conditions. It could be a muscle called the levator costorum, which is a muscle of your spine, a neck muscle, the iliocostalis cervicis muscle, spinal segmental sensitivity, or perhaps a neural issue coming from your neck at the lower cervical area."

"There are four things wrong?"

"No, but it is really hard to tell at this time which one is the issue. Right now, I could make a case for each one of them. Unfortunately, all of them are active. It is a little bit like a riot. Even though there are many people yelling and screaming, only about 15% of the participants actually know what they are yelling about. The rest are yelling because EVERYBODY is yelling. Muscles can be like that. In the next session or two, it should be clear what the real problem is. First, we deal with all of them. We need to quiet the riot."

Indeed, the next session was very different. The tissue itself felt much clearer; it was as though the fog had cleared and the underlying tissue restriction felt much more obvious. Instead of four possible issues, it seemed much more likely to be the levator costorum or the iliocostalis cervicis muscle.

S was very encouraged after the first two sessions. She was so encouraged, she mentioned the idea of going off her medication.

"I am a little uncomfortable with that," I admitted. "You should talk to your doctor about this. One possibility is to taper this very slowly. I'd like to know what your doctor thinks of that idea."

Indeed, her doctor thought the idea of easing down her medication was a good idea and suggested a protocol for tapering that seemed excellent. She had tried going off her meds in the past, but the pain always returned, coming back with a vengeance. It would often take several weeks to recover, even after she resumed taking the medication. She did not relish the idea of doing that again.

In the next two sessions, her tissue became clearer and clearer -- that is the only way I know how to describe it. I could now feel very tiny tissue texture abnormalities that were previously overshadowed by more superficial tension.

In this last session, both of us were marveling at how hyper-precise things had gotten; the slightest alteration in wrist position or angle was the difference between being "on it" or "off it." As I was again treating the iliocostalis cervicis, S remarked that she could feel that radiating up her neck.

"Show me where you feel that," I instructed.

"Right here," she said, pointing to the C6 area. "And that seems to radiate laterally a bit, too."

I immediately wondered if the posterior scalene might somehow play a role in this pain pattern. Examining the scalene in minute detail, I indeed found a tiny module that referred to the exact area of her spine where we had been treating the iliocostalis cervicis.

"Okay, this is just wild," I said, shaking my head at the irony. Check this out. The iliocostalis cervicis has a problem at the level of your shoulder blade, but it sends a neural input up to its superior attachment. Another muscle, the scalene, also attaches there. Some sort of spillover happens since they share the same attachment, and now the scalene is stirred up. It is well known that the scalene refers to, are you ready for this, the exact area we started with. What a feedback loop! How weird is that? Each one stirred up the other."

After disrupting the feedback loop, S was able to discontinue her use of the medication, and the pain only resurfaces about twice a year when she is under great stress. Since we know what to do, it has been an easy problem to manage. The rioters have gone home and are resting comfortably.

Real or Imagined?

Ahhhh.

As I was presenting to this class, every five minutes, another sigh would come. Like clockwork, another sigh would come again.

Ahhhh.

As a presenter, this is extremely irritating. Yet, the class didn't seem to notice. This was a group of students who had been together for several months. My assumption is that they had all heard this sound hundreds of times and did not even notice. I noticed. A lot.

Looking at C, the person emitting this sigh, her looks to me were uncomfortable. Her sigh was not one of relaxation, but clearly a pain behavior. Her looks to me while I was lecturing had the feel of, "If you really cared about pain relief, you'd stop talking and start treating me. Can't you see I'm hurting?"

These are uncomfortable moments. I only have limited time to be with a class, and my duties are quite clear. If I veer off into treatment of every participant, the road could go in many places far from my ascribed duties and may not be valuable to the class at large. It is hard to pursue two agendas. Usually, one accomplishes neither.

But, the sighs continued. Endlessly. At some point, I just could not take it anymore. At a time that worked, I did ask C about her pain. What a story it was.

C had helped a friend with disabilities get in and out of the bathtub. While helping her out of the tub, they both slipped, and C felt a sharp pain shoot through her back. What followed was a nightmare of pain and dysfunction. C had a profound distrust of doctors, but she finally succumbed. This was doubly difficult for her as she did not have insurance, making paying for medical care quite the challenge. The doctor prescribed muscle relaxers and anti-inflammatory meds for her, but C did not want to take them, nor could she afford the drugs anyway. She decided to tough it out, but the pain was winning. C had missed enough school that failing was a likely possibility, with more financial implications. She came to my seminar because she had to, but she was too consumed with her pain to focus on what I was teaching.

Deciding that this was educational for the class, I elected to treat C while the students observed. Since C was in too much pain to climb on a massage table, I had her sit in a chair while I addressed her back. Each time I barely touched the muscles of her back, she winced in pain. It was an effort to find ways to address her tissue at a level that did not create an exaggerated pain response. We struggled through this for about fifteen to twenty minutes, then stopped for fear of doing too much.

As the next morning came, students dutifully filed into class. I began to review material from yesterday, when breaking the morning silence was a loud and very audible Ahhhh. Oh no.

I did my best to push her sighs into the background, but I did wonder how she was doing after the work we did yesterday. I'm not proud of this, but at some level I did not want to ask, even though I wanted to know. If I ask and she is not better, then the day will be taken up with more treatment, as the end of the evening was last night. Alas, not asking became more obvious. I needed to address this.

"Can you tell me how you are today?" I asked, expecting the worst. Given the unchanged frequency of her sighs, I already knew the answer.

"Better," she replied. "I actually slept through the night for the first time in months."

I was stunned. "Can we check to see if your tissue is still as sensitive as it was last night," I inquired.

Obliging, C sat in a chair and we attempted to repeat what we did the night before. Her exaggerated reaction indicated it was still very tender. Yet, when I asked her if it was painful, her verbal response was a little ambiguous. We tried it again. Again, a very exaggerated response. Yet again, her verbal confirmation was unclear.

"Okay, let's do this one more time. Could you please just give me a one-word answer? Is what I am doing painful or not?" I instructed.

After her very marked reaction, I waited for the yes or no, but no answer came.

"I assume by your reaction, the tissue is still very sensitive and painful," I posited.

C shook her head no, which was confusing.

"It could be," she finally replied.

Oh my. Now I have my answer. This is a teaching moment for C and also for the rest of the class.

"I'd like to show you some research," I suggested. "I think you will find it interesting and very applicable to your situation."

What I showed C was some research done by Sawmoto and colleagues on pain and expectation. Researchers place a very uncomfortably hot object on a subject and observed which brain regions were activated. Next, they placed a slightly warm object on the subject and recorded that reaction. Cleverly, the next action was to tell the subject that the next object would again be very hot, like the first. In reality, the object was only warm, but the brain responded as if the object was uncomfortably hot. Scan number three looked like scan number one. In other words, you get what you expect.

Showing C the fMRI scans from the study as I explained it, I could see her mind processing the meaning of what I was sharing with her.

"Your brain cannot tell the anticipated pain from the actual pain, and neither can I. If every stimulus is perceived as a potential threat, your tissue is always under siege, even when no such threat exists. Discriminating real from imagined is essential to your recovery."

C returned to the seminar for the third and last day with a very difference countenance. Yes, there were occasional sighs, but much less frequent. At the end of the seminar, she shared how powerful discriminating real from imagined had been for her. Following up over the following weeks, her pain improved substantially, as did her attendance in class. I'm sure her future clients will benefit from her insight as well. What challenges us personally can make us better therapists.

Reclaiming the Body

"This is a very complicated situation. I just need to know whether you would be willing to take on something this unusual."

This was quite the phone call. My sense was that this woman was extremely hesitant, yet at the same time very desirous of an appointment. The more details she gave, the more interested I became. After assuring S that I appreciate and relish complex cases, S did make an appointment. I was anxious to meet her.

At our first meeting, S began to relay the details of her odyssey with pain after suffering a whiplash injury more than a year ago. The trepidation and fear in her voice were obvious, and her eyes were closely watching my body language, a signal that was hard to miss.

"My husband and I moved here from Israel about a year ago. This is all new for us: different job, different culture, a whole different life. Even the weather is not what I am used to. I have never seen snow, let alone driven in it. One day, while driving in a snowstorm, another car slammed into the rear of my vehicle. The impact caught me totally by surprise. At first, I did not feel severely injured, but my neck became more problematic about 48 hours later. For the next two months or so, my neck, shoulders and arms were very painful. I often had tingling sensations in both arms, which was very disturbing.

"The worst was yet to come. One day, I suddenly felt searing pain lower down in my back. Soon after, I felt tingling sensations in the front of both of my legs, which the doctors have told me is from a disc problem in my lower thoracic spine. That has persisted to this day. As time has gone on, I feel like my legs are wooden and stiff; like they do not belong to me. To make matters worse, about six months ago my family and I were in another accident, sort of."

"How do you 'sort of' have an accident?" I wondered out loud.

"My husband was driving and my two children were in the back seat. A car approached the intersection too quickly and was headed right towards my door. Judging the speed of the car, I thought that there was no way for them to stop in time. The car did hit us, but barely, the impact was almost imperceptible. There was hardly a mark on the passenger side door. My husband and children did not feel any impact at all and no one in either car was hurt, but I was in intense pain by the next day. The pain has been bad ever since. I can't explain why I hurt so much afterward; I think it was perhaps a form of post-traumatic stress."

"That is quite possible," I replied. "Even the medical definition of pain says as much -- an unpleasant sensory and emotional experience associated with actual *or potential* damage. The car didn't have to slam into you; just the potential trauma is enough to elicit the pain experience. The other three people in the car felt nothing afterward because the impending crash did not have the same meaning to them, as they did not have the same history going into the event. Your reaction is perfectly reasonable."

"Even though this is embarrassing, I need to confess how terrified I am to let you touch me," S confessed. "I am very afraid that treatment could make me worse, but I need to try something else because nothing has helped so far."

I assured S that I understood her fear and would do everything in my power to make her feel comfortable and in control of the process. "Where would you like to start? I asked.

"The most pressing complaint I have now is the lack of feeling in my legs, especially the right one, "she stated. "I'd like to start there."

I began with the lightest of touch, helping her to experience touch as a positive experience and not a threat. After some light fascial work, I applied lotion with gentle effleurage to her tolerance. After perhaps five minutes, I switched to the left leg with almost the same protocol, sensing her relaxing more deeply with each passing minute.

Returning to the right leg, I began to methodically trace each muscle of the lower extremity as though I was painting each muscle on a blank canvas. My goal was to provide clear sensory feedback to her somatosensory strip: the part of the brain that creates a topographic map of the body. That map is created in large part by sensory input, and S's sensory input had been quite compromised. In this application, touch is food for the nervous system, providing the brain with sensory data to help create the map based on *current*, rather than historical, information.

As I was finishing, S propped herself up on her elbows and looked at me with a big smile on her face. "I feel like I am reclaiming my body. I'm getting my legs back!"

When S returned for a second session, she reported that after returning home from the first session, she put on some music and began to dance, something she had not done for many months.

"It's like my body remembered how to move again, moving with joy instead of fear," she exclaimed.

If touch is food for the nervous system, then massage is a feast!

That Which Fires Together

"I have something new for you to address if you don't mind," said S. S is an amazing woman, having completed many marathons and several Ironman competitions. We have worked together for years, almost always on lower-body issues. People who do Ironman competitions have an abundance of lower-body issues!

"My neck is really becoming a problem. I can deal with it, but it is something I am almost always aware of now. I have been having headaches and general stiffness that is far greater than anything I can remember. I don't know if it is related, but I have been doing weight training this winter instead of putting in so many miles running or riding my bike. I thought it would be good for me to do something different."

"Do you notice any exercise where it is bothering you?" I asked.

"Not really, at least that I am aware of. My trainer seems very knowledgeable and keeps a close watch on my form. I don't feel immediate discomfort at the time, but it is hard to think that the weight training isn't involved, given the timing. The more involved I have been with weight training, the more my neck hurts. Yet, I don't feel it at the time. This is really perplexing," she shared.

"Are you doing any flexion movements, like the action of a situp?" I wondered.

"Yes, a few. He's pretty vigilant about the way I do them. Let me show you," she said, getting on the floor to show me the exercise.

She demonstrated one particular movement; while not my specialty, I couldn't see anything alarming. I did check the anterior muscles of her neck, starting with the sternocleidomastoid and the scalenes. Nothing seemed remarkably tender to her and the tissue texture seemed very compliant and soft. Since the anterior musculature was better than expected, I decided to explore the lateral aspects of the upper trapezius. This is a likely suspect for generalized tension, for the headaches she was experiencing, and often overloaded in weight training. The reality was much different than my speculation -- once again the tissue was remarkably supple, and she felt very little tenderness.

Having made the wrong call on several muscles, I decided to explore the semispinalis capitis with her in the supine position. Here I found quite a bit of tension and palpating this muscle replicated both her neck discomfort and headache symptoms. I had the feeling we were locking in on the cause of her discomfort, and she also felt that way. Reaching further down her paraspinal area with her in the supine position, I felt a large restriction at the upper thoracic vertebra. I was intending to palpate the semispinalis capitis, but the restriction I was feeling was horizontally oriented. Having her retract her scapula revealed that the restriction was in the middle trapezius.

What would explain this? It would be hard to make the case that the middle trapezius was the culprit since it does not typically create headaches or neck range of motion restrictions. The muscle was very tender but did not recreate her symptoms. Then what was its role?

I explained my dilemma to S and why the tension in the middle trapezius didn't make a lot of sense.

"The main job of the middle trapezius is to bring your shoulder blades together. If you squeeze them together, you will feel this muscle contract," I asserted.

I had left one hand under her upper thoracic area to palpate the middle trapezius, giving her proprioceptive feedback. By chance, I had left my other hand cradling her cervical area. When she brought her scapula into retraction, I felt her neck muscles, specifically the semispinalis capitis, tense. Whoa -- wait a minute!

"Can you pull your shoulder blades together without contracting your neck?" I inquired.

"I'll try," she replied as we repeated the shoulder squeeze. "Wow, I can feel myself contracting my neck, pushing against you every time I contract my shoulders. I know I should be able to squeeze my shoulders together without tensing my neck, but one action seems totally linked to the other."

There was a silence in the room as we both were processing the mechanics of the action. Suddenly, S jettisoned off the table in excitement.

"Wait, I think I might know how these actions got connected," she said enthusiastically. "Would this make sense?"

S then demonstrated an exercise where she was bending at the waist and bringing her outstretched arms into horizontal abduction. While this exercise is supposed to target her middle trapezius, it was also clear that her cervical extensors were tightening with every movement of her arms.

"My trainer loves this exercise," she said. "We do tons of them. He said this exercise is really important to enforce good posture."

"I think I understand the problem now," I stated. "There is a saying in neuroscience: 'That which fires together, wires together.' Each time you contract your neck erectors while simultaneously firing your middle trapezius, your brain learns to link the two actions together. It becomes like flipping a light switch: both bulbs come on even if you only wanted to illuminate just one.

"I remember reading a study where they asked subjects to do biceps curls with barbells that were a bit too heavy. As you might imagine, the subjects would thrust their pelvis to push the weight forward, as they could not lift it with the biceps alone. Later, the researchers gave the subjects very light weights and asked them to do biceps curls. The low back muscles fired! Why? Because doing it with heavy weights trained the back muscles to do so. You have trained your shoulder retractors and neck extensor muscles to fire simultaneously, and now we need to delink these actions in the same way you learned to link them in the first place."

S and I spent several minutes working on separating the two actions. I held my hand under her head and she tried time and time again to contract her middle trapezius without engaging her neck extensors. After many failures, she was able to successfully squeeze her shoulders together without tightening her neck. Once this relearning happened, both her shoulder and neck muscles softened substantially. We ended the session there.

I received a text from S two days later, stating how much better her neck felt. She realized her neck had been bothering her even more than she previously thought. Without the pain, she was able to sleep more soundly and completely than she had for weeks. Her trainer sounded very conscientious, and after she shares our experience with him, I think he will also appreciate a deeper meaning of the word "training."

The Audience and the Orchestra

My new client J has been struggling with hip pain for several months. Observing her gait, it was clear that her stride length was restricted, leading me to wonder about arthritic changes in the joint. Those fears were answered, as the radiology report found loss of space but only moderate joint degeneration.

"My doctor isn't sure what to do, as the joint looks better than my pain level reflects. The pain is really affecting my lifestyle and I just don't know what to do anymore," J confessed. "My doctor thought coming to see you might be helpful. I know the flexibility isn't good, but the hip is weak as well," she added.

"Show me how you know that," I replied.

From a seated position with her legs off the table, J tried to hip flex her right leg. It was clearly difficult, remarkably so compared to the left leg.

"Let me try something," I stated while moving to the other side of the table. Placing my hands on her back, I slowly began to explore the multifidi and quadratus lumborum muscles. I examined them in minute detail, changing length-tension relationships by altering flexion, extension, and lateral flexion movements of the lumbar spine. After releasing some exquisitely tender spots, I asked her to flex her hip again. She lifted her leg into much greater flexion and with far less effort.

"That's crazy," J exclaimed. "That seems like a parlor trick or something."

"No trick," I replied. "Just systems theory applied to anatomy. Lifting your leg is like pulling a drawbridge closed. The leg is the bridge, the chain is the muscle, but you need a wall to act as the anchor. That wall is your lumbar spine. Since your spine is moveable, the wall is made stable by the muscular contraction of your lower back muscles. If those muscles are compromised, the brain shuts down the movement as a protective mechanism. I treat your back, the brain senses that the wall seems stable, and now you can lift the leg. Cool, huh?"

"Amazing," she agreed. "So, this is a strength issue?"

"That's just one piece of the puzzle, not the whole picture. Let's explore more with you lying face down."

With J lying prone, I used the lower leg to create internal and external femoral rotation. The smaller muscles around the trochanter seemed reticent to allow the movement to happen.

Picking up the skeletal model with trochanteric heads, I put it on the table next to her and demonstrated femoral internal and external rotation. She thoughtfully watched the movement, observing the rotation of the trochanter in the acetabulum.

"Now, let's translate that into what you can feel," I instructed. While I rotated her femur, I had J put her hand over the joint to feel the motion.

"I can feel how some parts of the movement are not smooth. I can't seem to let go of those areas. Why is that?" she asked.

"This seemingly simple motion is actually very complex. There are multiple muscles around the hip, and for the motion to occur, each must let go in a very precise order. You could think of it like a symphony. Each instrument has an assigned role and must enter and exit at precise times. If the cello section won't lessen their volume when the second violins take up the theme, the sound goes from sublime to chaotic."

"Why do muscles do that?" J asked. "What makes some muscles go rogue and why do they stay that way?" she added.

"Great question; more research needs to be done to answer it. What I know is that my touch combined with your attention can help rewrite the software and push the muscular reset button."

Resuming the movements, J could feel her involuntary holding. "I want to let go, but how do I do that?" she implored.

"I don't mean to be coy, but you will figure it out. I'll keep doing the movement and you keep changing strategies until you discover how to let go." She was unsatisfied with my answer, which is understandable. It is, however, a really important point. Self-discovery is exactly that, self-directed learning.

Soon, the internal and external rotational movements became far easier. It was clear that something had changed.

"Somebody just figured this out," I teased. "The orchestra is playing better."

"Definitely," J agreed. "Do you know what the most amazing thing about this process is? I am feeling my own body, but at the same time, I am witnessing it. I feel like I don't have full control, but observing it changes it."

"An amazing process," I stated.

"What is really amazing is that I feel like I am part of the audience and part of the orchestra at the same time!"

The Map

"I think the pain is right in here," B said, pointing to the anterior thigh just in front of the trochanteric head. Shifting her seat in the chair, B continued to press into her anterior thigh, as if somehow she could not find what she was looking for. Without speaking, she continued to explore her thigh muscles.

Lifting up her buttock, she began pressing deeply to explore the posterior aspect of her left hip.

"Actually, maybe the pain is really coming from here," she stated. This statement was followed by more shifting and probing, then a very awkward silence as she realized that she had no idea where to direct my attention.

Standing up, B elaborated on her experience. "When I move, the left hip just does not feel like the right. I can turn easily and move from my right hip with total freedom. When I do the same on the left, it is less clear, and the movement is more restricted."

Watching B move, I was in awe. B is a world-renowned dancer and choreographer and moves with a sense of grace that one seldom sees in the general population. Her internal sense of restriction is so refined and sensitive that I could barely tell a difference visually. More important than my visual assessment is what B experienced. Her expert sense of her own body, refined through thousands of hours of training, told her that something about the left side is a little off. My job was to help her rediscover her left hip.

Asking B to lie supine on the table, I took her hip through a range of motion in flexion, internal and external rotation. Not surprisingly, the range was stellar. Doing the same on the right, I could find no perceptible difference between the two sides. Her experience, however, was that the left side moved less freely than the right. Feeling no perceptible difference in range, it was clear to me as to what approach to pursue. Reaching for the spine and pelvis model, I had B sit up while we reviewed the anatomy of the hip. Showing her the movements of flexion, extension, internal and external rotation, we reviewed the actions of the joint and the muscular implications during each motion. I could see her visualizing each motion in her own body as we were demonstrating them on the anatomical model.

Proceeding back to the table, I had B lie prone. Bending her knee at 90 degrees, I used her lower leg to rotate her femoral head internally and externally. I placed the hip model next to the table so periodically B could glance at it to remind herself of exactly the mechanisms of movement.

"That is so cool," B exclaimed. "I can visualize and feel the movement now, something I was having trouble doing before. In other parts of my body, I have an internal picture of how the joint moves. For whatever reason, I could not do that with my left hip. How strange."

Moving to her right hip, I replicated the same internal and external rotational movements that we did on the left. B confirmed that for whatever reason, she could easily connect with the movements on that hip, having a very clear internal representation of the movements I was doing.

"I, too, find this process fascinating," I shared with her. "It is a very important principle that is often overlooked. Each of us has a map of our body in the brain, and that map can dictate our experience and perceptions. There are many examples of severe disturbances of the map, but someone like yourself, with a finely tuned movement system, will notice things that the general population will not. The combination of my precise palpations and your observing the movement in the skeleton rewrites and clarifies the map. That clarification should then also translate into a change in the experience of movement as well. That is what you have been experiencing. Let's do some more!"

This time, instead of moving her leg into internal and external rotation, I stabilized her femur and moved her hips and low back in a rocking motion. Before I could say anything, B broke out in laughter.

"Okay, now you are moving the hip in reverse, a sort of hip motion through no motion. The socket moves around the ball, instead of the ball moving around in the socket. Very tricky!" B remarked, with a knowing smile.

"Busted," I admitted, while we both shared a good laugh.

After getting up slowly from the table, B began to dance around the room.

"I am fully present in my hip again," she said. "I can feel it, I can see it, and my hip is part of me again. I am going from here into the studio to work on this new piece I'm creating."

One of the most gratifying aspects of working with a client like B is the knowledge that she will turn this shared experience into a dance that will thrill and inspire audiences worldwide. In some small way, I got to play a part in it.

The Power of Knowledge

I greeted N in the waiting room, happy to see this energetic woman in her seventies back in my office; I had not seen her for many months.

"What brings you in today?", I asked. "How is your back doing?"

"My back is doing fine; it has been quite good for a long time now. I am here today because of my left shoulder. After five months of pain, I am ready for it to end."

"Five months? Wow, I'd say that's long enough to be in pain. Was there an event that initiated this pain, or did it escalate slowly over time?" I queried. (I did not fully share with her what I was also thinking. If I helped her back that much, and she was in a bad state, why would she wait five months to see me to address her shoulder? Some mysteries remain unsolved.)

"I can't think of any specific incident, other than painting the two back bedrooms in my house. After a month of pain, I went to see my doctor. She diagnosed it as impingement syndrome and gave me some medication, which makes me tired and doesn't help very much. After a few weeks, she also referred me to physical therapy. I have been doing the exercises, but they haven't helped. The pain is really starting to wear me down. Is this something you have seen before and can you help me?"

"I have seen this many times, and there is every reason to think that precise soft-tissue work can help," I replied. "First, I'd like to check something."

Putting her humerus into full internal rotation, I passively lifted her arm into forward flexion. As soon as we went past ninety degrees, it recreated the pain in her shoulder. This test confirms that impingement syndrome is very likely. At that point, I asked her to lie on her side on my table, so that I might palpate the supraspinatus.

N voiced a question just before I began. "I want to ask a question before I forget. My husband and I have always slept in the same position for years. Unfortunately, that means that I sleep on my left shoulder, which is the one that hurts. I think sleeping on it makes it worse but changing to lying on my right side messes up our sleeping routine. Is it bad to sleep on my left side?"

Before I opened my mouth to give her an answer that seemed obvious, I thought about a much bigger concept that might be far more important.

"Has anyone explained to you what Impingement Syndrome actually is?"

I asked. "No, not really," she replied.

I am not sure how long I hesitated in replying to her, but the implications of her statement cascaded me into a sea of thoughts. You, the reader, might make the case that previous health care providers did explain impingement to her, and she didn't understand or remember, but this is a *very* bright woman who could not explain it to me now. How can a person know what to do or what not to do without understanding the nature of the condition itself? I have seen countless clients who have been given a diagnosis of some sort and yet possess no real understanding of the mechanics of how that translates into real life. In our rush to perform a treatment, we neglect to form a deep understanding of the problem. The more completely we understand a problem, the more likely we are to create effective solutions.

"Let's spend a few minutes with my skeletal model before we get on the table," I said, inviting her to the skeletal model next to my desk. "Do you see this deep space?" I said, pointing to the supraspinatus fossa. "That is where a muscle called the supraspinatus is located. It attaches at the top of this bone, called the greater tubercle of the humerus. Notice how the tendon has to pass under this boney shelf. If there is too little room, the tendon gets squished, and therefore inflamed."

"What would cause it to get squished?" she asked.

"There are two common reasons, a fall or repeated small traumas. Watch this," I said as I raised the humerus into abduction. "Anytime your upper arm is above ninety degrees, you compress the available space. Or, if you fall forward with your arms outstretched, the humerus is jammed up into the socket and that smashes the tendon and the bursa."

"Uh-oh," she remarked.

"Uh-oh?" I questioned, widening my eyes in curiosity.

"I did have a little fall before the pain started. I started painting the bedrooms within days of the fall, which might have been the last straw. I was planning on painting the kitchen next. I bet using a brush and roller overhead isn't going to be a good thing for my shoulder right now."

"You've got that right. Plus, what happens to the available space for the joint when you lie on that side?" I questioned.

"Lots of compression," she said. "No wonder that position hurts. My husband and I will just have to adjust to a different sleeping position. Lying on my left side isn't going to work for the foreseeable future."

"I think that is a good idea. You guys can figure it out, but lying on your left side is a problem," I stated. "Let's take a look at a few muscles that may be playing a role in this problem."

I explored her supraspinatus and deltoid muscles, finding some tenderness, but not overwhelmingly so. The teres minor was another story, however. It was very tender, and this muscle can play an important role in impingement. Due to its angle, the teres minor can help pull the humeral head downward during abduction, which decreases compression. Research data also shows that the pectoralis minor, when shortened, also can decrease the glenohumeral space. This muscle was rather tight on N, and we spent some time addressing it.

Since impingement is a condition of intrajoint inflammation and sensitivity caused by trauma, it was not reasonable for N to arise from the treatment table pain-free. She was indeed more comfortable, but the underlying condition would take a bit of time to resolve. The hands-on work could speed up the healing process; the functional anatomy knowledge would keep her from doing anything to further insult it.

After N left, I thought about how differently she must feel about her shoulder pain. No longer was shoulder impingement simply a name; she now understood what was happening, why it happened, and what not to do. That knowledge alone is powerful healing.

Chapter Three: Client Education

*"For the body/brain, it isn't just about
what you feel. It is also largely about the
meaning you assign to what you feel."*

"So, tell me again, when did this happen?" I asked.

"About seven weeks ago. I did see a doctor, but there was nothing broken or torn. The joint was very swollen and, as you can see, it still looks different than the other side," she said, pointing to her right index finger metacarpophalangeal (MCP) joint. "The doctor said I could splint it temporarily, but she wouldn't necessarily recommend that approach. Her suggestion was to move it as much as possible, which is what I have done. The problem is that I cannot move it completely and the finger just doesn't feel right."

"What was the mechanism of the injury?" I asked.

She looked sheepish as she described being in a hurry at a conference she was coordinating. While running to the bathroom, she jammed her hand against the toilet paper holder.

"Wow, we need a new story. We'll get to that later," I couldn't help interjecting. Returning to the issue I said, "Show me what movements you can or cannot do."

She made a fist, revealing full flexion range of her index finger. Index finger extension, however, was limited in relationship to the other fingers of her right hand and also to the non-involved left hand.

"Mostly, I notice that I do not have strength in this finger. When I try to press on anything, such as a spray bottle, my finger is really weak. I've painfully learned how much I use my index finger," she revealed.

I reviewed the game plan. "There are three areas of concern: The finger flexors, the extensors, and the ligaments at the joint itself. What I am going to do is reason through each of these possibilities until we understand where the problem lies.

You have full flexion range, but not strength. That means that the extensor muscles will allow the motion. Your extension is reduced, which could be caused by flexor shortness or extensor weakness.

Another possibility that would explain both is something called arthrokinetic inhibition. In this model, an injury to the joint sends a message to the muscles that cross it to not contract fully. This is a protective mechanism for the joint. When muscles span a joint and contract fully, it increases joint pressure. Sensing that increased intrajoint pressure may be dangerous, the brain shuts down the contractile capacity of the muscles to protect the joint. Muscles can heal readily, but joint injuries can last a lifetime. Therefore, the brain will always sacrifice muscles to protect the joint."

At this point, I began by carefully examining both the flexor digitorum superficialis and profundus muscle and tendon associated with the index finger. While she had full range of motion, there were some surprisingly tender areas in the muscle belly.

"Wow. That really is tender. Is it really tight?" she asked.

"Not tight, but injured and inhibited. Muscles essentially do one thing, and that is to contract. When they are injured, they do that one thing less well, which you experience as a weakness. My goal here is not to increase range, but to increase strength. What about this muscle?" I asked, palpating the extensor indicis.

"That is even worse," she replied. "What is that?"

"This muscle contracts to extend your finger backward. It looks like it isn't the flexors being too tight to allow the extension to happen, but that this extensor muscle is too weak to pull the finger backward."

"So, both of these muscles were inhibited by an injury to the joint," she summarized. "The flexor muscle is weak enough that pushing on a bottle of hairspray is hard. The extensor muscle is too weak to pull the finger backward to the same distance as the other fingers."

"Exactly. The system is very functional in the short term. The joint injury sends a message to the muscles to shut down to protect further injury to the joint itself. Unfortunately, when the joint was no longer at risk, the muscles didn't get the memo that it was now safe to resume full activity. This could go on indefinitely without treatment."

For the next twenty minutes, I alternated treating the extensor and flexor muscles of the index finger using moderately deep unidirectional friction movements in the direction of the muscle fiber. I also did cross-fiber friction of the ligaments at the metacarpophalangeal joint.

When she returned a week later, the swelling had visibly decreased, and extension was just shy of normal.

"The biggest difference I notice is that I find myself using this finger during daily activities. It is much stronger," she stated elatedly.

"I'm thrilled it is much better. Now, one more thing. I just want to be very clear about how you injured your hand. When you dove in front of the

oncoming car, reaching out with your right hand to corral the child who had
just wandered out into the street . . ."

Availability Error

"You're kidding! Seven?" I remarked with astonishment.

"Yep, seven softball games in one day," H replied with pride.

"How the heck does that happen?" I asked. "Is this the softball version of a marathon? Or some sort of court-ordered punishment?"

"No," H laughed. "Just a big tournament with a bunch of old guys. Most of us come from great distances, so we have to play all the games during one weekend."

Events like this fly in the face of physiological principles. In running, there is the 10% rule; you never increase your mileage more than 10% a week. Doing more than that increases your risk of injury. The human body does not do well with spikes of activity. For instance, I love to cross-country ski. Snow is very intermittent in Champaign, IL; when it snows, I want to get out there and ski for hours. Not a good idea, since I might not have skied for a year. The same is true for people who fly to a warm climate and play endless rounds of golf in three or four days, then wonder why they hurt.

This principle applies to massage therapy as well. New therapists in my office are the most likely to have hand and arm issues. A good part of the reason, beyond efficient mechanics, is an erratic schedule. We try to be careful with them for the first year, not allowing them to see too many people in one day. After a year or so, they, like the therapists in my office who have been there for many years, can see people all day long without injury. It's a consistency thing.

Regarding H, I needed to know more about his injury.

"Was there a specific incident that initiated your left thigh pain?"

"I was running the bases, trying to stretch a single into a double when I tweaked my right ankle pretty seriously. I was able to run on it, or perhaps I should say limp on it, for the rest of that game. Unfortunately, that was game five and we had two more to play. By the end of game seven, I felt this pain in my thigh. It disappeared after a few days but resurfaced with a vengeance later."

I just stared at H, trying to process these details without getting distracted by the fact that this guy is 67 and can kick my butt from here to Maine and back again. (That, coupled with the fact that I have a knack for stretching a double into a single.)

"What happens if you lift your leg? Any pain when you do that?" I queried.

As H lifted his leg (hip flexion with no knee extension), I happened to put my hand over the rectus femoris muscle belly. What I felt was a remarkable protrusion of muscle tissue right in the muscle belly. I have seldom felt such a pronounced muscle projection such as this. My first thought was of several clients who have torn their long head of the biceps brachii. As the biceps muscle retracts, it looks like "Popeye", leaving the person with what looks like a massive biceps. Outlining the muscle projection with my fingers, I knew I was on to something big.

"Is this painful?" I asked, knowing that it would be, but wanting to confirm the fact.

"Nope," H replied with indifference.

Pressing harder right into the epicenter of the muscle bulge (how's that for trying to prove myself correct?), I asked H again if my pressure created discomfort.

"Nope, nothing" he responded indifferently.

I looked at H with confusion. "It is thigh pain that we are addressing?"

"Yes, it really hurts sometimes. My sleep is quite often interrupted."

"Does your thigh hurt during activity?" I asked.

"No, I do wind sprints and distance runs without any pain at all. If I do leg extensions on a machine, there is no pain during that exercise either. The only time my leg hurts is at rest."

Why in the world can he run with no pain if the problem is a tear in his rectus femoris muscle? That is exactly when I had my "aha" moment, realizing that I was looking at this whole problem incorrectly. There is a principle in logic called availability error; the tendency to choose the most obvious answer with what is most available to us. The explanations readily available to us can be recent examples of other people with similar symptoms, or, in this case, something attention-getting like a big muscle bulge commanding my attention. The moment I saw the bulge, I assumed, whatever his pain, that a tear had to be part of the problem. In essence, I wanted the problem to fit my answer, instead of the other way around. I decided to start over, taking the tear totally out of the equation.

"Is your leg in pain now, just resting on the table?"

"No, as long as I am on my back, my leg is fine. What really sets it off is if I turn to lie on that side. Lying on it can create pain that lasts for hours."

"How about this muscle? Is this sensitive?" I asked, pressing into his vastus lateralis. H almost levitated off the table.

"I'll take that as a yes," I quipped.

"Holy cow! I can't believe how painful that is," H exclaimed with a strangely satisfied tone of voice. Interestingly, I could see that he was happy to have someone validate his pain. My pressure recreated his mysterious pain, something that no one else, even he, had done previously. Even H had assumed the bulge was the source of his problem.

For the next twenty minutes, I treated his vastus lateralis, gluteus medius, gluteus minimus, and tensor fascia latae slowly and methodically. The tenderness abated substantially, and he volunteered to be diligent about stretching his thigh over the next few days.

I called H about a week later to check his progress. His leg had seldom hurt. He had even awakened to find himself lying on his left side.

"What about the lump?" H asked. "Will it go away?"

"Perhaps a better question is, should you care?" I responded.

"If the pain is gone, I guess not," he admitted.

Lighter Socks

"I can't believe how much my back hurts," said M, an active young man in his mid-thirties.

"If I bend over, even a little, it really grabs, like it is going into a spasm or something. At its worst, it can take my breath away. My doctor said it is a muscle spasm, but man, this feels like a lot more than just a muscle problem," M remarked.

M's comment is a really interesting phenomenon both in the world of pain science and in our personal experience. It is an understandable but misguided assumption that the severity of pain indicates the severity of the problem. His assumption is that muscular problems are not so serious, therefore the intense pain he is experiencing could not be muscular in nature. There are at least two problems with that assumption. First, when researchers explore which conditions cause the most pain, muscular spasm is right up there, after kidney stones and childbirth. Second, there are cancers that are lethal, yet cause no pain whatsoever. I felt I needed to address his statement.

"I understand why you think that, but actually, a muscle spasm can be one of the worst pains you can experience," I assured him.

"But this hurts too much to be just muscle. I think something really serious must be wrong," M asserted.

"That's the funny thing about pain. We would like to think that serious problems hurt worse than less serious ones, but that just isn't true. A paper cut on your tongue can be devastating, yet a deadly cancer may have no symptoms at all. There just isn't a linear relationship between the danger and severity of pain."

"That's what my doctor told me yesterday, but I have a hard time believing that to be true. But if you and my doc are right that this pain is muscular, I don't ever want to feel it again. Ever. You have to tell me what movement to avoid. Whatever the trigger was, I don't want to do it again."

"Have you been doing anything out of the ordinary?" I asked.

"Not really. I did carry big boxes of tax receipts up into the attic, but that was almost a week ago. I also helped my son and daughter-in-law move into their new house, but just for a day last week. Oh yeah, then I changed the plumbing under our bathroom sink, which turned into a nightmare. A two-hour job turned into a whole weekend of work. I was fine until yesterday when I bent over to put on my socks and my back seized up."

"I think I know the remedy," I answered thoughtfully. "You need lighter socks."

M just stared at me for a second, not knowing whether to grimace at a bad joke or whether I was actually serious.

"Lighter socks, really?" M questioned.

"Okay, not really. What you want is to be able to identify a singular movement that caused your back spasm. In reality, there isn't one event, but a perfect storm, where bending over to put on your socks was simply the last straw," I explained. "Most often, pain like yours is often the result of a cumulative process of tissue insult. None of the individual stresses could cause this pain, but the cumulative effect is devastating. Moving the boxes, helping your son move, or fixing the sink -- none of these alone would likely have caused this. Collectively, they caught up to you big time."

"OK, I get your point," he admitted. "But there must be some specific movement that caused this in the first place. There has to be some movement I am doing incorrectly. I don't want to live in fear of moving the wrong way and being in pain again," M stated.

Even though there are certainly times when specific movements are irritating and should be avoided, I strongly felt that M's case wasn't one of them. What I found fascinating was his intense desire to identify a singular cause. This desire also opens a fascinating window into both pain science and human behavior. Just so that I follow the norms of science when speaking of human behavioral science, we begin with rats!

Research studies of reward behavior (press a lever, get food for instance) demonstrate that the chemical that mediates the reward centers of the brain is dopamine. Dopamine is a fascinating and yet dangerous chemical; surges of dopamine are intensely satisfying and pleasurable. How is it dangerous? These same reward centers of the brain are also probably where addictions reside. Ingest cocaine, and dopamine levels skyrocket. Worse yet, after the high, the resting levels are lower than before the fix. This necessitates a greater dose, and a vicious cycle ensues. Rats that have access to pressing a lever to flood their system with dopamine will do that endlessly, foregoing all else.

Let's now imagine a slightly different scenario, one in which randomness is introduced. Let's say that the rat is in his cage, just having a normal day, when BOOM, a big reward is bestowed. What does the rat brain do? It looks for a reasonable explanation. One can imagine an internal dialogue (assuming rats have an internal dialogue): "Okay, I just got a reward. Let's see. What did I just do? I need to do that again. What was it?"

Studies of the stress response reveal the same thing. Reward or punish a rat in a predictable way, and stress levels are negligible. Reward or punish them randomly, and stress levels skyrocket. Why? In rats and humans, we seek order and predictability. I did this, therefore this happened. If no reasonable explanation is available, one will be provided. We make one up.

Thinking of all of this in the background and finding a way to get my point across, I offered up a crazy idea.

"Okay then, the answer involves $750!" I said as M stared in disbelief.

"Here is the deal; I am going to see you for two to three sessions in the coming days. In less than two weeks, I predict that your back will feel substantially better, perhaps completely recovered. In about a month or so, you will have forgotten all about this pain episode. Sometime in the next six months, I am going to call you at exactly 6:12 in the morning. When you answer the phone, I am going to inform you that today is the day of reckoning. Your task on that day is to recreate this back pain within a twenty-four period. If you can do that, I will pay you $750. Cash. If you are unable to recreate the pain, then you owe me $750. Sound like a plan?"

"No way," M responded. "I don't think there is any way I could do that. That's crazy."

"I'm pretty sure you couldn't do it either," I replied. "So sure, I'd bet $750 on it. My point is that you couldn't recreate this back pain if you were paid handsomely to make it happen. There is no need to live in fear of possibly repeating some mysterious motion that would send your back into a spasm. A more reasonable approach is to resume your normal daily activities as much as possible. The fear of moving in the wrong way may be more detrimental than any particular movement itself.

The overwhelming odds are that your back pain is the sum total of multiple factors, the act of bending over to put on your socks was simply the straw that broke the camel's back. Probably, if you take out any one of those factors, your back would not have spasmed putting on your socks. When you are dancing on the edge of the precipice, even a slight breeze can send you over the cliff. It took the sum total of all those goofy factors to create your present circumstance. That's not likely to happen again anytime soon. Over-protective guarding of your back may do more harm than good."

I could see M's face soften as his fear eased. Three sessions later, his back was doing just fine. I checked in with him with follow-up calls at three and six weeks; his back was doing splendidly. I never did make that phone call at 6:12 in the morning; I don't think I needed to! I think he got the point.

Maybe İf You Just Press Harder

"My levator scapula is killing me," she exclaimed. With that opening sentence, it was clear that my client, Mrs. M, had some background in anatomy. The funny thing is, these self-assessments are seldom correct (including my own!).

"Tell me more about that," I invited.

"I am a physical therapist, and at the hospital I am often pushing and pulling on patients from awkward positions. There often isn't an ergonomic way to move them, and I'm sure that is what started this pain. For the last three weeks, the area of my scapula near the medial angle has been really angry. At first it was intermittent; now it is my constant companion."

"May I check a few things first before we jump right into treatment?" I asked.

I had Mrs. M sit in front of me while I passively moved her neck checking her range of motion. Since the right side of her neck was the problem, I expected some limitation in left lateral flexion. To my surprise, I could not perceive any restriction or even a hint of hesitation on her part. I tested lateral flexion again, but this time to the right. Again, no hint of pain or limitation. Repeating left lateral flexion again, this time I put her neck in flexion to prestretch her levator scapula. There was still no limitation in left lateral flexion. As the final movement, I raised her right arm overhead, which rotates the scapula into upward rotation. Since the levator scapula helps to create downward scapular rotation, this arm position (plus left lateral cervical flexion) creates maximal stretch on the levator scapula. Still, she felt nothing.

"I don't feel much of a stretch, but it's pretty tight back there, isn't it?" M inquired.

I smiled and nodded with no verbal response. To be honest, I find these questions quite awkward. Mrs. M was looking for confirmation and validation, yet that isn't what I found with my assessment. She knows what she feels, but the reason for her experience is probably not what she thinks it is. For me to say that so early in the session is quite risky; it could easily be interpreted as invalidating her perception and refuting her assessment of the source. That is not a good decision if I wish to create therapeutic alliance with a client. On the other hand, I want to tell the truth about what I find. I decided to go in a different direction.

"Let's explore this on the table. Could you lie face up? Let's see what we find in the tissue," I directed.

With Mrs. M in the supine position, I put the right scapula in a slightly elevated and protracted position, exposing the levator scapula attachment at the upper angle of the scapula.

Pressing quite firmly into the tissue, Mrs. M gave no reaction.

"Is this tender?" I asked. "This is where the levator scapula muscle attaches to the scapula."

"Maybe if you press harder," Mrs. M responded.

"Let me try something first," I replied.

Changing the angle of my wrist, I directed my pressure to the second and third rib, rather than the scapula itself. Mrs. M winced in pain and shot me a look of astonishment.

"Oh, my goodness, that is super tender," exclaimed Mrs. M. "I don't think I can take that much pressure. Does the levator scapula attach there as well?"

"Actually, it's a completely different muscle and there is an important lesson here. May I show you something?"

Placing my finger on her forehead, I demonstrated the amount of pressure I was using on her rib, which was just over two pounds of pressure.

"You're kidding. That's all the pressure you were using? It felt like more than three times that much," she said incredulously.

"When I was on that first area, do you remember saying it might be tender if I just pushed harder? I was using almost three times the pressure at that point and it still wasn't tender. Isn't that amazing?"

"Why would that be?" she asked.

"In my experience, when people ask me to press with an inordinate amount of pressure, I'm simply in the wrong place. Pressing harder won't improve the situation. Touch is a form of communication, and the amount of pressure I am using is much like volume in verbal communication. If you don't understand what I'm saying, I doubt that you would want me to say the same thing louder. You'd probably ask me to say it differently. Pressing really hard is analogous to yelling. If what you say is communicated clearly, you shouldn't have to yell. That's hard on everybody. In this setting, it's hard on the client as well as the therapist. Great results depend on precision, not pressure."

"I am assuming that the second place was a different muscle. What was that?" asked Mrs. M.

"Welcome to the serratus posterior superior," I replied. "Nasty little guy, that one. Shall we continue?"

What followed was very focused, gentle, and thorough work on her serratus posterior superior. I have seen her for three follow-up sessions, and her symptoms are 95% better. We had excellent results, she is thrilled to be symptom-free, and best of all, no yelling!

Perception Deception

"I know you are some sort of specialist in massage therapy. I have seen other massage therapists in the past, but they did more general approaches. I figure your approach will be deeper and much more painful, probably more than other massages I've had. I am willing to do that to get rid of this tightness."

"That's quite an opening line," I remember thinking to myself. My new client, Ms. D, had presented herself to my office on this afternoon, and typically my office manager gives me a heads-up about the nature of the appointment. In this case, I had none and needed much more information about the goals for the appointment. But what an opening line! (Not one I hear very often.) In the mind of my new client, Ms. D, effectiveness and focus translated into more discomfort *during* the treatment, not simply better results. I find that rather astonishing; how did she get these ideas? Some of it could be self-generated, but much of it is likely to have come from other massage therapists. Either way, I had a challenge in front of me.

"What is our goal here?" I inquired. "What is the one thing that you are looking for me to help you with?"

"I'd like you to release the tension in my Upper Trapezius. The tension in both of my upper traps is constant and very annoying. It is a sensation that is with me always. If I could release the traps, I'd feel so much better. We do have one little problem that I should let you know if you need to see me for more than two sessions," she stated.

"What's that?" I asked, curious as to where this was going.

"I am scheduled for surgery on my ulnar nerve about three weeks from now. We have until then to work on my traps, after which I will be out of commission for several weeks. I was hoping to get some relief before the surgery," she admitted.

"Whoa. This is a bit of a revelation. I'd like to hear more about this first if you don't mind. Tell me more about why the surgery was scheduled."

"Several months ago, I started having problems with my fingers," she said, pointing to her little finger and ring finger on her left hand. "These fingers feel weird."

"When you say weird, what do you mean exactly? Numb? Painful?"

"I guess I mean that they often feel numb and kind of fat. They don't feel like my other fingers. It has been this way at a low level for almost two years, getting progressively worse over the last several months. I have been going to yoga class and getting massages regularly, but the problem continues to worsen. I saw a neurologist and she did a nerve conduction test which showed my ulnar nerve has some sort of a problem. In the surgery, the plan is to move the ulnar nerve from the cubital tunnel to somewhere else, but I'm not sure where."

"Usually, the nerve is placed under the forearm flexors, which must be cut and then reattached to the common flexor tendon. It's a pretty extensive surgery," I stated.

"They said as much. The recovery will take several weeks. I am already gearing up for what that will mean for my life. It won't be easy. That's why I was hoping you could help me with my shoulders. I'm worried that the stress of the surgery will make the shoulders even worse and I have enough to deal with already."

"I certainly do understand that," I replied. "I'd like to help you as much as I possibly can. Moreover, it might be possible that these two situations, the shoulder tightness and the nerve issues, are related. If we help one, it might help the other."

"That's nice," she said. "But, I am already scheduled for surgery. The doctor thinks that moving the nerve is the only way to solve the problem. It seems like a done deal. Is there really a chance to avoid the surgery?" she inquired.

"Let's wait on that for now. First, let me look at a few things. Since no obvious trauma started this, there must be some low-level trauma irritating the nerve. Would you stand up and let me look at your structure?"

Ms. D stood up and I placed my hands on the spine of her scapula to assess shoulder height. Standing back, I looked carefully at her structural presentation. Tall and rather slim, she presented as a woman with a long and rather elegant neck. With that as a clue, I looked closely at her scapular alignment. As I suspected, the lower apex of her scapula was much closer to her thoracic spine than the upper angle of the scapula. This was true bilaterally, meaning both scapulae were significantly downwardly rotated. Interestingly, this gives the illusion of having a long neck. More interesting, as the scapulae are in a downwardly rotated position, it places the upper trapezius in a lengthened, stretch-weakened position. Since the muscle is held in a lengthened position, the stretch receptors are always firing. Perhaps this explained why she perceived the upper trapezius to be 'tight'.

"Everyone keeps telling me to keep my shoulders back and down," she admitted. "They tell me that doing so might help the nerve symptoms in my left hand. I must not be doing it often enough to make a difference because the neural symptoms haven't improved at all. If you have any tricks to help me remember to drop my shoulders, I'd love to hear them."

"This might be the opening I need," I thought to myself.

"First, can we try something? I want to you to sense the feeling in your left ring and little finger in your left hand. Now, pull your shoulders back (posteriorly) and down and keep them there. Let's keep them there for about another fifteen or twenty seconds. Does the position of your shoulders change what you feel in your hands?"

"That's really weird. I can feel my hand go numb the longer I hold my shoulders back and down. Am I doing something wrong?"

"Well, first and foremost, I wouldn't suggest pulling your shoulders back and down anymore. Your shoulders are already downwardly rotated, which compresses the clavicle against the first rib. The nerve that serves your fingers goes between the clavicle and your first rib. When you pull your shoulders back and down, you compress these nerves."

I walked Miss D over to the skeletal model in my office and showed her the relevant anatomy. Talking about this is helpful, but nothing replaces being able to see and touch the skeleton to increase deep understanding.

"I have something I'd like to propose to you," I offered. "This is a little out of the ordinary, but I think I can help you with both your shoulders and your nerve issue in your left hand. In fact, I think they are really connected, as you just experienced. The position of your shoulders may indeed be the irritant that creates your neural problem. I'd like you to contact your surgeon. I know him quite well, and he is an excellent doctor. Ask him if the surgery is time- sensitive and, if it isn't, I am wondering if both you and he would agree to delay the surgery for up to two months. If your symptoms disappear, then you will be spared both the surgery and a long recovery process. If I am unsuccessful, you owe me nothing; there is no charge for all the sessions that we will do. Timewise, you may need to budget for up to ten sessions. If your doctor agrees to this, would you be willing to consider trying this first?" I inquired.

"Um, I'll certainly consider it. Do you really think you can help with both issues? Isn't surgery inevitable?"

"There are no guarantees to success, only that I will give this effort my absolute best. But, I think there is a strong chance this may help. If I'm right, you are going to save a lot of money, time, and suffering. If I'm wrong, you will only be out the time. Fair enough?"

Ms. D did indeed contact her doctor. While he wasn't completely thrilled about the delay, he did state that the surgery was in no way time-sensitive. Waiting for another two months or so wouldn't make a difference. As she stated, his response was, "Knock yourself out, but we will still, in all likelihood, do the surgery. What Doug will do can't make the condition worse, but is unlikely to help you, either."

Game on.

One of my first hurdles in the treatment process was to help Ms. D understand why her upper traps weren't really the source of her troubles. Since she had focused on her experience of upper trapezius discomfort for so long, this was not going to be easy. Plus, I needed to redirect her thinking in a way that did also not invalidate her experience.

"Can I have you stand up? I would like to try something with you regarding your shoulders," I asked. Having her stand in a normal stance, I asked her to sense what she feels in her upper trapezius.

"It feels tight!" she said emphatically, "I always feel tension there."

"The sensation of tightness may actually be deceiving. Try this; take an inventory of your trapezius tightness and slowly bring your shoulders back and down like you did earlier. Don't move your shoulders as much as before, perhaps half the effort you did previously. What do you feel in the upper trapezius area?"

It took Ms. D about thirty seconds or so to answer.

"I feel even more tension in my traps now," she said, looking perplexed.

I asked her to return to her normal stance and then repeat the downward rotation of her scapulae one more time. The result was still the same.

"Watch what happens when I do this," I suggested. I gently lifted her shoulders to rotate her scapulae, putting them into a more neutral position. I saw a slightly perplexed smile come over her face.

"That feels really good," she remarked. "It feels like that position takes all the tension away."

Taking Ms. D back to the full skeletal model in my office, I placed a flex band over the attachments of the upper trapezius.

"When your shoulder blades downwardly rotate, the upper trapezius muscle is pulled taut, like the way this rubber band is being stretched. If you run your finger over this band, it feels stiff and is under tension. That stiffness is not true tightness, but too much stretch. Getting it to relax won't work, as it needs to shorten, not lengthen. Do you see how that applies to why you feel what you feel?"

"Oh my gosh, that is really interesting," Ms. D exclaimed. "My perception may have deceived me. My massage therapists and I were mistaking tautness for tightness, trying to lengthen and relax an already overstretched muscle."

"Right you are. I doubt many therapists can feel the difference between tightness and tautness by palpation alone. Hands can feel tissue texture differences, but only knowledge and understanding can correctly interpret the meaning of what is felt. Good therapy not only treats soft tissue but helps you, the client, understand what you feel and why."

"Where do we go from here?" Ms. D inquired, ready to get started. "What muscles need to be treated to help reposition my shoulder blades?"

Ms. D was exactly correct in her thinking. Essential knowledge for the therapist is the ability to take what is observed and turn that into a treatment protocol. If the scapulae are downwardly rotated, the therapist must know which muscles are responsible for that position. Who are the downward rotators of the scapula? The major muscles involved are the rhomboids, latissimus dorsi, and levator scapula. All of these can be easily accessed in the side-lying position.

When Ms. D was side-lying, the full amount of the restriction was evident in the simple act of taking the scapula into elevation and upward rotation. As I gently tried to move the scapula superiorly, the resistance was obvious. Ms. D also noticed the tension and resistance in the movements.

"Am I letting you do that movement? I feel like I am having trouble letting go and allowing you to move my shoulder. It doesn't hurt or anything, but I seem to be holding it tense."

"Yes, you are holding a bit, but that's understandable. This kind of tension is controlled by a part of your nervous system that isn't under conscious control. The only way to change it is to observe it dispassionately."

Over time, as I kept moving her scapula, she indeed found a way to let it go. Allowing me to move it into elevation was clearly the most difficult motion for her.

All of the muscles that produce downward rotation were quite sensitive to touch; the most sensitive of all was the latissimus dorsi.

In the end, it took about five sessions for the scapular muscles to release; there was a very visible change in her presentation. Her shoulders were no longer sloping downwards. More importantly, the neural symptoms in her ulnar nerve faded away.

Ms. D did return to see her physician after we finished our work, wanting his opinion about the prospective surgery. His response?

"Really? Do you think I'd do surgery on someone with no symptoms?" He was admittedly quite impressed and surprised. Think of the money saved by her insurance company and the lengthy recovery she did not have to endure. Score one for the home team.

"I brought some things for you to read," said my client.

"Whoa, you certainly did," I thought to myself. L had a stack of paper about a half inch thick, organized chronologically.

"I thought you might want to see these physician reports, physical therapy notes, and let's see, what else," as his voice trailed off looking through the papers.

"Before I do that, could you tell me what brings you here?" I asked.

"My right hip hurts. Nothing has helped, and several people recommended that I see you," he admitted.

"Could you tell me in your own words what you feel and what other people have done?"

"One of these reports describes the injection," L stated, looking through the papers.

"Injection?" I asked.

"Yes, a steroid injection in the hip about six months ago. It didn't help, so we decided that the pain wasn't coming from my hip. An X-ray of my spine showed a narrowing of the disc space, so we thought the hip pain was coming from my back. An MRI showed a possible disc issue which was extremely discouraging."

"The vast majority of people with no back pain also show disc abnormalities on an MRI," I countered. "Perhaps you are one of those people, where it shows up on the MRI, but it isn't clinically relevant."

L struggled to process this information, trying to relegate the MRI image with the idea that it might not matter. The image clearly had a powerful effect on his perception of the problem.

"Maybe that's true," L admitted. "After the MRI, I had a back injection and there was no improvement in my hip. We tried a second injection in a different place and still my hip was unchanged. I then saw an orthopedist, but he did not think that back surgery was in order. He recommended physical therapy using the McKenzie Method® for my back, which I did for three months without results. I guess that is why I am here."

"It seems to me that everyone thinks your hip pain originates from your back," I stated. "Another possibility is that your hip pain is actually coming from your hip."

"But the X-rays looked fine and the injection into my hip didn't help," countered L.

"True, but that doesn't rule out problems with the muscles around the hip. You have had great people treat your back, but if that was the source, your hip pain would be better. Let's take a different tack and see what happens. It's worth a try, as nothing else has worked so far."

Showing me his pain, L pointed to the lateral aspect of his hip. He stated that occasionally the pain runs down his leg, even below his knee. With that symptom presentation, it made sense as to why people thought the source of the pain might be coming from his back. It was very similar to a typical sciatic nerve presentation.

"Does this look familiar?" I said, showing L a referral chart for the gluteus minimus.

"It sure does," he affirmed.

Having L lie on his left side, I took his right leg into adduction. The moment I lowered his leg towards the table, his pelvis also moved caudally, showing restricted range of motion of the gluteus maximus, gluteus medius, and quite possibly the gluteus minimus. As I began pressing firmly on the gluteus medius and minimus, L's eyes widened.

"Wow is that tender!" he exclaimed. "Is it supposed to hurt like that?"

"Nope. Notice what happens if I move about 2 cm posterior," I said. Barely changing my hand position, I pressed into the tissue again.

"That doesn't hurt at all," he replied. "Why is that?"

"While there are multiple muscles in your hip, the problem is likely to be one or two of them, and only in very small selected areas of those muscles. The whole problem is hyper-precise. Miss those tiny areas and the results won't be positive." It takes patience and skill to locate and then treat these very small injured areas.

Moving anteriorly and closer to the trochanter, I found an exquisitely sensitive spot. L's facial expression changed immediately.

"That shoots right down my leg!" he exclaimed. "What the heck? Why is that?"

"There are two issues here, what and why. The *what* part is clear; if I press exactly that spot, you feel it down the leg. The *why* part is not clear; how this referral happens is not well understood. On the other hand, we used aspirin for decades without understanding how it worked. Not understanding the mechanism doesn't prevent you from using something effectively. The key is replication. I have treated scores of people with this same symptom, and they no longer have the pain radiating down the leg. And just to be clear, this was not a temporary fix; years later, the symptoms have still not returned. This is true not just for a few people, but more than one hundred. In the end, results matter," I stated, making sure he understood.

Making subtle changes to the position of L's leg allowed me to examine his gluteus medius and minimus in multiple length-tension relationships. Changing the angle of entry and the direction of my pressure, I examined the abductor complex in minute detail. I retested L's adduction capability after twenty minutes of treatment; his range had improved significantly. Standing up, L noticed an immediate difference in his mobility. He also perceived an increase in strength, as though his leg was now part of a more solid base.

"I'm surprised that something so simple was so effective," shared L.

"Simple, but not easy," I replied. "As a mentor of mine pointed out, these are different concepts. Telling the truth is simple, but not often easy. Finding areas of tissue disruption is also a simple concept but is seldom easy."

"I know one thing. Next time I hurt, I am doing this first," L shared.

Thus, a new advocate for the power of massage therapy left my office.

The Goldilocks Principle

"I don't really like massage very much."

"You what? Seriously, who doesn't like a massage?" I looked at J with astonishment. J seemed like a very bright guy, full of life and energy, a barista at a coffee shop I had visited for the last three days. He had wondered why I was there three days in a row, yet I had never been there before. I explained that I was teaching continuing education for massage therapists in his community and dropped into his store for coffee before the training. That's why he responded with his comment about massage, which completely surprised me.

The moment I responded, I hesitated at the quickness of my response. There are many reasons that people might not get a massage; some of them a physical condition, and some a deeply personal, emotional reason which would make massage uncomfortable. I hoped I did not tread on sensitive territory. Just as I was lost in worrying about my brash response, he continued.

"I just don't really enjoy getting a massage. I am sure what you are teaching is helpful, but I have had about six massages and I am done trying."

This was getting more interesting with each comment.

"Was it the therapist, the environment, or the massage itself? What was so unpleasant?"

"My experience has been that the therapist either uses pressure so light that it doesn't feel like anything is happening or that the pressure is so great that it feels like he/she is trying to kill me. There doesn't seem to be a happy medium."

"Do you mention this to the therapist? Do they adjust the pressure?"

"When I have tried to do that, the therapist inevitably defends the particular approach being used. Nothing changes. It just isn't worth spending more money trying to find someone who uses the right amount of pressure for me."

His words felt like it took the wind out of me. How sad is that? Here is a bright guy who doesn't value the field of massage therapy because he can't find someone to use the right pressure.

My friend and colleague Christopher Sovereign recently referenced the Goldilocks Principle, a scientific principle that I have been thinking about ever since. If you remember the children's story, Goldilocks found the extremes of things in the house unsatisfactory, while only one was "just right". In biomedicine, too much or too little of the same substance does not produce the desired effect. Just about everything in life follows this principle. Too much or too little, and the results are lacking. Success lies within defined margins, not outside of it.

In the world of massage, the Goldilocks Principle is certainly in play. With regard to pressure, there is an amount that is clearly "just right" for the recipient. Finding that perfect level of pressure is no small task, one that can be thwarted in at least two ways, one internal and one external.

Internal Processes: If the therapist has a preference for lighter or deeper pressure when he/she is the recipient, that same therapist tends to assume everyone likes what feels good to them. During a training, I will often be demonstrating a technique, only to see one of the therapists in the audience cringing. When I ask why, they say that the technique must be really uncomfortable. When I ask the person I to who I am demonstrating the technique if it is painful, they often tell me that it is not. For instance, if a therapist finds any work on their SCM uncomfortable, the assumption is that so do all their clients. Massive assumption.

External processes: Finding the "just right" pressure implies that the client will give the therapist honest and accurate feedback. Truthfully, this does not happen very often, leaving the therapist to rely on his/her perception. (When people have complained about incorrect pressure at my office, the client almost always states they assumed the therapist knew what they were doing, and this was the way massage was supposed to feel. Since they had no experience with massage, they relied on the therapist's judgment.) This leaves the therapist flying blind. It is hard to succeed without feedback.

It is important to remember, however, that in this case, J did give the therapist feedback and the therapists he saw tried to educate him as to why that particular amount of pressure was the "right" way for him. That's really sad.

Pressure alone is not the essence of massage; there are numerous other variables also subject to the Goldilocks Principle. The perfect amount of pressure in the wrong place will not be effective. In a session with my last client, ascertaining the precise location of his tissue restriction was an elaborate process.

"Try pressing a bit harder," he stated. "Nope, that isn't exactly it. Close but not quite. Try angling your wrist a bit. Nope, the other way. Better, but not yet. Wait, let me try moving my leg just a bit forward and see if that helps. Oh, that's better. Perhaps if I rotate just a little…whoa! Right there! Don't move a millimeter!"

Throughout that whole process, I simply followed his directions because he clearly knows the exact spot that will replicate the all-too-familiar pain in his hip better than I could ever possibly hope to. My job is to know the possible suspects, his to help me target the exact one that replicates his discomfort. The look of satisfaction on his face when we hit the "just right" spot with "just right" pressure said it all. So did the results.

Pressure and location are only two factors of massage affected by the Goldilocks Principle; two others are client communication and environment. The therapist must establish rapport with the client by asking questions and being engaged from the moment he/she greets the client. Being too quiet can be interpreted by the client as aloofness and disinterest, while talking too much can be seriously distracting to the massage experience. The massage environment is also affected by the Goldilocks Principle; professional but inviting, temperature that is not too hot, not too cold, music that is as ignorable as it is interesting, and a schedule that runs on time but never feels rushed.

With all the factors that have to intersect to create a wonderful experience for our clients, it is no small task to get it "just right". There is great satisfaction in the effort, however; the grail is in the seeking, not the cup.

Unhappy

"Would you mind giving this person a call? She wanted to speak to the owner."

As the owner of a massage therapy clinic with many therapists, a request like this from my front office staff ramps up my heart rate a few notches. Seldom do people want to speak to me because they want to share what a fabulous experience they had with one of my staff. More often, as you might imagine, something has gone wrong and the person wants to express his/her displeasure. These conversations are never easy, but I sincerely appreciate that the person took the time to give me feedback.

Dialing the number with a sense of anticipation, I was a bit surprised by the very pleasant voice belonging to someone who had visited my clinic a few days earlier. After explaining who I was, Ms. R, sounding a bit embarrassed, explained her frustration.

"I didn't want to say anything to you, but my mom bought me a gift certificate for the session. When she asked how it was, I told her how disappointed I was. She just wouldn't let up, insisting that I call you. She has been going to your office for years and loves the place and thought you should know about my experience. It's not that I am complaining or that I want to get the therapist in trouble, but the session wasn't at all what I expected. I have never had a massage before, and I was really looking forward to it. After all those high expectations, I was really disappointed with the session. I don't mean to be a complainer; I just want you to know I am very disappointed."

"First, you shouldn't apologize at all for expressing what you feel. If we as an organization failed you, I need to know. I cannot correct a problem that I don't know about. Tell me what was disappointing with the session."

"It is not so much that the massage itself was a problem, just that the session was really incomplete," she relayed.

"Incomplete? How do you mean that?" I asked.

"I mean that the therapist spent all her time working with my neck, shoulders, and upper body. The massage in that area was great and really needed. The problem is, those are the only areas she worked. She did not massage my legs at all, just a little work on my back and hips. I'd say that 90% of the session was focused on my upper body."

"Oh, I see. You were hoping for something quite different from what you got, so of course, you were disappointed," I restated.

At this point, I couldn't help but wonder how the goals for the session could be so far from what the client wanted. This is very uncharacteristic of my staff, but everyone can have a bad day or make an occasional bad choice. I decided to pursue it further.

"Did the therapist sit down with you and discuss what your goals for the session were? Did she take the time to ask you what, if any, areas were of concern?"

"Yes, she did sit down with me at the beginning and asked me where I was feeling tension and stress. I told her about the headaches I was having, and how they have been an almost daily occurrence for the last two weeks. I think they are coming from my shoulders, both of which are extremely tense. Also, the area between my shoulder blades has been driving me nuts. If I sit for any length of time, I get this burning pain and my job requires me to sit most of the time. Between the aching in my shoulders and the headaches, life has been pretty miserable. That is why I was looking forward to the massage so much. I have even been missing work because of the neck and shoulder issue. Even when I am at my desk, I find it hard to concentrate because of the discomfort."

Before I could respond, Ms. R interjected.

"Uh-oh. I just realized that everything I complained to the therapist about was right where she worked. I didn't think about it, but she did exactly what I asked, or at least what I complained about. I just never thought about it until just I heard myself tell you what I told her."

"Did the massage help those areas she addressed? Are your shoulders better and have you had a headache in the last two days?"

"My shoulders are less tense and, come to think about it, I haven't had a headache either. I am feeling really embarrassed right now because it seems I got exactly what I asked for, even though I expected something different. It's just that my image of massage was a whole-body session, with maybe just a tad more emphasis on an area of tension. I am not even sure where I got that idea, maybe from the movies or something. I just didn't think a massage could be focused like that."

"The practice of massage is wide-ranging, from more general relaxation to highly specific problem-solving. While my therapists can do both, our specialty is in problem-solving, which is what the therapist did based on your description. We could have perhaps done a better job of clarification of goals, and I'd like you to come in again for a free session just to relax. Make sure you tell the therapist that you want a relaxing full body session. It is also important for you to know that you can change your mind at any point in the session. If the therapist is concentrating on your neck and you feel it is resolved, feel free to direct her elsewhere. You get to drive!"

As I hung up the phone, I kept thinking about assumptions and the model of understanding of the word 'massage.' When people hear 'massage therapy', what comes to mind? I recently voiced that same question to a class of massage therapy students who were visiting my office. Inquiring about their own model of understanding of 'massage therapy', the first student responded with the word 'sleep.' The second student's response was 'physical therapy.' That's about as wide a range as you can get, and these are massage therapy students! If we as a profession see this field with such a wide variance, is it any wonder the public perception is all over the board as well? I do not pretend to have an answer, but this problem will probably haunt the profession for a long time to come.

In the meantime, massage therapists must clarify not only the client's stated goals, but also unstated pre-conceptions or assumptions that could affect potential outcomes. Sometimes, that's the hardest work of all.

Whiplash

"I am grateful; the accident could have been so much worse. I was very sore, but that did not start until about two days after the collision. The soreness kind of surprised me, as I didn't feel much of anything right after the crash, just thankful we were not hurt more seriously. I wasn't going more than a few miles per hour, but it still could have been much worse."

I then asked M, an energetic woman whose accident had occurred about a week previous, to describe what happened.

"I was in a parking lot and was backing out to leave. I had my head rotated over my right shoulder, but I didn't see the car backing out across from me until right at the last moment. He didn't see me and backed right into my car, giving me quite a jolt. I suppose my neck would have been better off if I had just relaxed, but I tensed at the moment of impact as I saw him coming toward me but could not stop in time."

"Actually, you did just the right thing and that is probably why your neck is as doing relatively well after the accident. It's not like you really had a choice in how the accident happened, but the fact that you saw it coming was likely a very good thing. The outcomes when you know the impact is coming are far better than if you don't."

M looked at me with surprise. "Seriously? I thought it was better if you were completely relaxed at the point of impact."

"The research data shows exactly the opposite. When you tense, your muscles protect the ligaments and the delicate structures around the joint capsule from massive compression and/or shear force. The muscle tissue does suffer in the process of tightening to protect you, but muscles heal far more quickly than ligaments or joints. The body will always sacrifice muscles to protect deeper structures. That is the wisdom of the body; protect the joint even if the muscle takes the brunt of the injury."

"What about the idea that people who are drunk seem to survive terrible crashes? That seems to conflict with what you just told me."

"Actually, a whiplash such as yours, and a typical accident involving a drunk driver are two very different scenarios. The whiplash process is essentially over in less than one second, about .6 seconds. An accident where an intoxicated person drives off the road and rolls the car over several times is a multi-second event. It is known that in multi-second traumas, being relaxed is generally a distinct advantage. This is also true in accidents like falling down some stairs, stumbling out in the woods, or other events that take a few seconds to unfold. Slipping on ice, however, can happen so fast it almost approximates the speed of whiplash, and therefore can often create nasty injuries that last. In a motor vehicle whiplash, being unaware and therefore completely relaxed is definitely a liability. Numerous studies have shown this to be true."

"Wow, I guess I did the right thing without knowing, or, at least my body knew what to do! Do you have an idea why the left side of my neck is so sore?"

"You were looking over your right shoulder, correct? If the head is turned to the right and the impact shoves the torso forward, the neck will be pushed into additional right rotation and your neck will go into extreme extension. If the neck is turned to the right and you want to stop it from going too far, you

---

"Tighten the muscles that turn the head to the left!" blurted out M. "You'd also tighten muscles that stop the head from going backward, too!" exclaimed M with a big smile on her face. "That's why the left side of my neck hurt the next day; it stopped my head from going too far."

"You are exactly correct! Great reasoning skills -- I'm impressed! Shall we examine the muscles to see which is most involved?" I asked.

After M was supine on the table, I checked her range of motion in right and left cervical rotation. She had a very slight restriction, albeit slightly less range to the right than to the left. To check any involvement on the right side, I put her into right rotation with a little extension and compressed her neck slightly. This created no discomfort at all, a good sign that no facet inflammation resulted from the impact. The only discomfort M felt was on the left side of her neck just anterior to the trapezius. As I palpated the posterior scalene, I could feel the muscle tighten in response to my pressure. The muscle was over-reactive to length changes; hyper-responsive to both passive lengthening and passive shortening. Just as I was ready to zero in on the posterior scalene, she spoke up.

"Have you ever had the feeling that your arm was too heavy like it was tired or something? My left arm feels different than my right, and it goes down to my thumb and behind my shoulder blade, too. Maybe you could check my mid-back out before the end of the session," she suggested.

"I will, but first let me try something," I replied.

As I carefully searched the posterior scalene, the moment I hit the right spot, M's eyes widened. One spot replicated all her symptoms: the pain on the left when turning right, the pain down her arm, and the pain near her scapular border. The excitement on her face was captivating, a childlike enthusiasm for solving the puzzle at hand. Showing her the scalene referral pattern, I could see her relief as she understood what she felt and why. Her understanding of the mechanics of the injury, the muscle involvement, and the seemingly random symptoms now coalesced into a clear picture. I'd bet that facilitating her understanding was at least as important as the treatment I did to the scalene muscle! In the end, treatment of the scalenes was amazingly effective. The cervical rotation was improved and the midscapular pain disappeared as well. There was another side effect as well; I was a little more cautious when backing my car out of the parking space when I left the office that evening!

Chapter Four: Clinical Reasoning

"System problems require system solutions."

Classic Thoracic Outlet Syndrome, That Wasn't.

"I am so grateful! I can't believe it is still better."

These kind words greeted me from the enthusiastic woman tagging my luggage as I was checking into the airport ticket counter at my local airport. It is always a bit difficult when seeing a person out of context; it took me a moment to place her and the condition with which she first presented about three years ago. Her enthusiastic greeting revealed that she had been symptom-free ever since the treatment.

M had been a client at an advanced training at my office which focused on the relationship of soft tissue and symptoms of neural entrapment. She presented with sensations of numbness and upper extremity pain which she had been experiencing for several months before her visit. M had been to her physician and numerous other health care providers, to no avail. My co-instructor for this seminar, Seth Will, had asked M to describe her symptoms to help us better grasp the problem.

"I have pain and numbness in my right arm and hand. As I remember, there was no specific incident that started it, just something I increasingly noticed as time went on. The numbness isn't quite the same as friends who have had carpal tunnel syndrome; it feels more like a glove that dulls my whole hand. I often feel it all the way up my arm and sometimes even into my middle back. The pain is often worse upon arising but gets better during the day. Sometimes my hand feels cold and the whole arm just feels heavier than the other side. The discomfort has never been intolerable, but it is a serious annoyance that interferes with my life and my job. I work for an airline at the ticket counter. It has been particularly busy in the last year; staffing cuts eliminated the person who used to help me with baggage. That means I am handling a lot of bags during the day, as well as ticketing passengers. As you might expect, many of the bags can be pretty heavy. People often stuff them so that they are just under the weight limit. Slinging the bags all day long can be very taxing."

For the benefit of the seminar participants, Seth demonstrated very precise neural testing for each major upper extremity nerve that might possibly be implicated. Not surprisingly, none of the tests pointed to a specific nerve as the likely culprit. What would account for her neural symptoms but yet no specific nerve seems to be compromised?

By the look we exchanged initially, both Seth and I were pretty sure that we were looking at classic Thoracic Outlet Syndrome. While this seemed really promising as it fit with her symptoms, none of the common tests for Thoracic Outlet Syndrome were positive either. What else might explain her symptoms?

When a client presents with neural symptoms similar to Thoracic Outlet Syndrome and concomitant midback pain, the scalene muscles are often implicated. We proceeded to thoroughly examine her scalene muscles and unfortunately, we found nothing very remarkable. Again, this was surprising as the scalene muscles seemed like such a perfect fit. If all the pieces do not fit, it isn't it. Don't try to make it fit.

Since nothing we had done so far seemed helpful, Seth and I decided to regroup and start over. (Not a hard decision to make when you are failing miserably.) We were clearly missing something important that might take us in a different direction. But what?

Thinking about the mechanics of moving luggage gave me an idea. "Would you please lie face down on the table? I'd like to check something."

After M was situated on the table, I began to slowly press against the spinous processes in her thoracic spine. As I approached the lateral aspect of the spinous process of T4, she reacted strongly.

"That's it. When you press there, I feel it right down my arm and into my hand. That makes all the symptoms come back at once."

As soon as she said this, the source of her problem became clear. A few years previously, I had also seen someone who presented with neural symptoms that I found perplexing (truthfully, any neural symptom was pretty perplexing to me a few years ago). One person, in particular, was dramatically and immediately helped when I treated her thoracic spine. Most remarkably, this discovery was completely accidental. I was as surprised as the client. (It's probably not the greatest marketing strategy to act dumbfounded when the person tells you how much better they are, but I have a lousy poker face.)

That first client's improvement was so dramatic, I resolved to research why in the world treatment of the thoracic spine was so effective. When I need insight, I go to the research world to learn from the experience of others. I soon discovered that other clinicians had also discovered the source of atypical upper extremity neural symptoms to be in the thoracic spine. This condition is called T4 syndrome, which is slightly misleading since the source of the problem could be any of the upper thoracic vertebrae from T2-T5. The sympathetic nerves emanating from T2-T5 affect the upper extremity, and there is a close relationship between the segmental nerves and the sympathetic nerve afferents. The sympathetic chain also is strongly affected by problems at the costovertebral joints. The palpatory confirmation of T4 syndrome is a highly sensitive spinous process at the site of entrapment, which must recreate presenting symptoms.

Seth and I decided to treat the muscles affecting the costotransverse junction such as the levator costorum, rotatores longus and brevis, and iliocostalis thoracis. With M, the immediate results were a lessening, but not a complete cessation, of her symptoms. We called to check on her two days later; symptoms had continued to decrease incrementally each day. Since the training was over and we felt she was moving in the right direction, I did not continue to communicate with her.

Having not heard from her since then, it was extremely gratifying to know that her symptoms disappeared completely about a week after the session and had not returned in three years. Lessening symptoms temporarily is one thing but sustaining that improvement for three years is a different matter. She is symptom-free and profoundly grateful to have her life back. As evidenced by the way she effortlessly tossed my luggage onto the conveyor belt, work hasn't been a problem either!

One Client: Three Very Important Lessons

Mrs. M came to my office complaining of pain in her knee, which had undergone replacement two years previous. Most people I've seen with knee replacements do very well, but Mrs. M was still having pain and she was walking with a very obvious limp. Her story has three important lessons for all of us in health care. Let's examine each of them individually.

Lesson One: Invalidation. When she went to her orthopedist (the doctor who did the replacement) complaining of pain, he largely ignored her concerns. She, who had never had a knee replacement, did not know what to expect. He, having done many, should have given her some guidance. Each time she brought up her discomfort, he was dismissive. At first, she thought that perhaps this was normal and that the pain would lessen. Talking with her friends who had also had a knee replacement, none of them had her level of pain that long after the surgery. She was now very frustrated.

After a year and a half of pain, the doctor decided to refer her to physical therapy. The physical therapist agreed that her knee pain was unusual and a cause for concern. Voicing that concern to her doctor at her next appointment, he explained that the knee pain couldn't be coming from the replacement. There must be something else going on. Really? When the presenting symptoms do not fit neatly in the paradigm of the provider, the provider often questions the validity of the patient's concerns. Mrs. M felt as if the doctor did not hear her or refused to believe that the new knee could still be painful after all this time.

Much of the premise of my book "The Mystery of Pain" revolves around invalidation. Patients can be invalidated by friends and family who do not understand chronic pain, or by healthcare providers like Mrs. M's doctor. I had my own experience of invalidation many years ago, and it is one I have never forgotten.

I had been doing massage for perhaps a year or two and I wanted to experience Rolfing, both for the experience and also to correct my postural imbalances. My pelvis was markedly unlevel and that seemed connected to other conditions, such as low back pain and neck issues. Saving up every penny I could muster, I drove to Chicago (three hours away) to get ten sessions of structural bodywork. I don't know how I afforded it, as I was dirt poor at the time. However, I did it; getting Rolfed was a big deal, financially and emotionally. I was new to this field and full of enthusiasm and hope.

Looking at the pictures after the tenth session, the asymmetry in my pelvis and shoulders was relatively unchanged. This was pretty devastating, as I had so much hope, not just for my own results but for the promise of the power of bodywork. Instead of questioning why the results weren't there and what he might change to improve the outcome, the Rolfer explained that my lack of structural change was probably because I wasn't emotionally ready to accept such a change. Not only had I spent every dime I had without seeing the changes I hoped, but this person, in a position of power, was telling me that I was at fault. Needless to say, this was devastating to me. I felt like a complete failure. About 15 years later, I discovered that I had a rather significant anatomically short leg. Short of a miraculous event, my anatomically short leg probably isn't going to get any longer via soft tissue work. I am very careful now to stress to clients that if I fail to help them, it says everything about me and very little about them. If I can't help, there is an answer out there somewhere. Keep looking.

Lesson Two: Clinical relevance. Assuming that the knee pain must be coming from another source (because it could not be coming from the replacement), the doctor ordered an MRI of Mrs. M's back. Not surprisingly, moderate disc pathology was found. The doctor decided disc pathology was the real source of her knee pain. When Mrs. M explained that she almost never had back pain and saw no connection in daily life that would substantiate this assertion, the doctor was unmoved. He prescribed an epidural injection in her back to address her knee pain. This was not something Mrs. M was excited about doing; she just wanted someone to treat her knee. The doctor refused any further treatment, even refusing to see her again unless she had the epidural.

That her lumbar MRI showed moderate disc pathology is not surprising; in a landmark study published by Jensen et al in the *New England Journal of Medicine* in 1994, the majority of people who have *never* experienced back pain have serious disc pathologies on their MRI scans. This is not to say disc pathology does not exist or is not a possible source of pain. It does, however, call into question the idea that disc pathology equates to back pain since asymptomatic people have the same pathology. Scientifically, this is not defensible. Whether the issue is a radiologist using a diagnostic image or a massage therapist finding sensitive soft tissue with her hands, the most challenging question for every practitioner is whether or not what is found is truly relevant to the person's presenting pain. One can find stuff wrong, but it does not mean that what you find is connected to the symptom. "What" is easy. "Why" is not.

Mrs. M decided not to see her doctor again, as each time she did was another study in frustration. She also did not do the injection into her spine, as this would have been expensive for her and did not seem connected to her knee problem. She decided to see me for several sessions to discover if soft tissue therapy could help her. We did something remarkable: I worked on her knee!

Lesson Three: Neural patterning. After a few treatments, Mrs. M had a substantial increase in pain-free flexion of the knee. She was thrilled with the progress we had made. After summarizing which structures I treated, why, and what the game plan was for our next session, she stood up to leave my treatment room. As she walked toward my door, I noticed her limp was still quite pronounced. I asked her if putting weight on her knee was painful. She enthusiastically replied there was no pain when doing so. I found this quite perplexing. Taking her hand, I asked her gradually to put weight on the side of the replacement. Finding it comfortable, we kept increasing how much weight she put on her knee. (This probably looked like a ballroom dance move we repeated over and over.) We achieved complete midstance (full weight) without pain. When she questioned why we were doing this, I remarked how she was still visibly limping, yet she stated that she had no pain in weight-bearing or walking. A look of epiphany came over her face as she realized she was limping completely out of habit, not out of pain. The knee was better, but the brain hadn't gotten the memo!

Mrs. M's story is a powerful mix of three lessons very relevant for all of us. It challenges us to listen carefully and validate our client's experience. We must be thoughtful about deciding whether anything that we find in our palpation or assessment is connected to the presenting symptom. Lastly, we must remember that creating the potential for better movement is just that, potential. That potential must be realized by helping the client change his/her movement patterns or referring to a practitioner who specializes in doing just that.

"It hurts right here," said K, pointing to a spot right just above her left PSIS. "It has been uncomfortable but not debilitating for many weeks, but it does affect me when I play."

K is an elite level collegiate tennis player, one of the best in the nation. My office is in Champaign, IL, which is the home of the University of Illinois. The U. of I. was the host for the NCAA National Tennis Championships. Teams from all around the country came to compete for the national title. When the trainer for the U. of I. gave my name to one of the teams, the word spread through the tournament. My office was insanely busy seeing these players, and while it was an intense schedule, it was also an amazing opportunity to see high-level athletes like K. I have worked with many amazing athletes over the years, but these tennis players were special, and K was among the best of the best. Her movement patterns and body awareness were superb, which makes working with athletes of her caliber a joy.

"Is there any simple movement that you can do now that recreates the pain?" I asked.

"Actually, I feel it as a slight pull or nagging sensation when I simply bend forward at the waist. I only feel it on the left side when I bend straight forward."

I observed her flexing forward and we established an exact angle of flexion that initiated the discomfort. Noting the exact angle where discomfort happens will help us track progress; the goal is either greater motion or, at the very least, minimal to no discomfort at the same initial angle of flexion.

In my mind, I ran through possible suspects that included muscles such as the multifidi, erector spinae, and the quadratus lumborum. The long dorsal ligament and the iliolumbar ligament were also possible suspects, as was the SI joint. I had K lie on her side and began by treating the multifidi first. Starting on the surface of the sacrum, I treated the multifidi thoroughly all through the lumbar spine, finding only a few tender areas. After I finished, I had her stand up to re-audit the original movement.

"No real change," she admitted.

"Okay, I know who it isn't!" I pronounced. "Let's explore another muscle, called the quadratus lumborum. Please have a seat on this stool." Sitting behind her, I carefully examined all three sections of the quadratus. Unfortunately, no spot recreated her pain, even though some points were sensitive. Asking her to stand up, we reassessed forward flexion again. I could tell by her facial expression that it had not improved.

"Sorry," she said. "No change."

"No need to be sorry," I replied. "Let's examine another possible cause. Please lie again on your right side." At this point, I decided to palpate her iliolumbar ligament, which was located near the epicenter of her pain. Challenging the ligament did not elicit the presenting symptom, however. I moved my finger slightly inferior to be just medial to the PSIS and found a sensitive point. Pressing medially on the ASIS, I was hoping that the sensitivity on the point near the PSIS would decrease. (Pressing medially on the ASIS decompresses the SI joint.) No such luck.

Asking her to stand up, she again flexed forward. Doing so, she looked up at me with an apologetic face. "No need to say anything, I can see that didn't work, either. Just so you know, this isn't over until you flex forward without discomfort. No excuses. You're not leaving until this thing is better!" I insisted, half joking but determined to figure this out.

"You're relentless!" she said teasingly. "Just like me," she added.

"I'm sure that is true," I said. "What makes both of us excel is an unyielding commitment to results. No matter how hard the journey or how long it takes, we embrace the struggle, because that's where learning takes place." As our eyes met, I saw in her someone who has known great success and learned from countless failures along the way. She displayed a sense of confidence and wisdom that was quite impressive for someone so young.

"Wait, let's try this," I suggested, breaking the moment. "What happens if you flex forward from a seated position?"

"There isn't any pain at all," she stated, sounding surprised.

"Okay, what would account for that?" I asked myself, thinking out loud. "Stand up again and let me try something."

This time I cupped my hand around her sacrum, guiding it forward as she flexed her spine. Unfortunately, there was no change in the pain. Positioning both my hands on her pelvis, I guided it anterior as she flexed.

"Wow," she exclaimed. "That totally eliminates the pain. Amazing!"

"Here is what I think is happening," I explained. "There are muscles that create a posterior pull on your hips as you flex your spine forward. If the hips don't have enough motion, the spine is forced to do too much. Let's treat those muscles and see what happens."

Placing her side-lying again, I did fascial work over the posterior thigh and specifically treated the adductor magnus and biceps femoris.

K rose from the table to check progress. I knew immediately from her smile that the results were positive. There was still a slight pull but at a much greater range.

Her trainer called me the following day, thrilled with K's progress. For me, I kept thinking about how a personal commitment to excellence allows us to recognize and celebrate that same commitment in others, no matter what their discipline. Luckily, as therapists, giving our best enables those we treat to perform at their best. What an honor!

Results Matter

"I[MC4] can take a lot of pain, but man, this thing really hurts. If I could cry, I would."

Looking at my new client, there was no doubt in my mind that he could indeed take a lot of pain. B was a solidly built guy in his 50's, and every aspect of his presence conveyed a sense of toughness. Dressed in heavy work clothes, B was my first appointment of the day. He had come right from work, having worked another all-night twelve-hour shift.

"My leg really hurts," B explained. "It started several months ago, and I thought it would just get better on its own, but it never did. It has been getting to be more and more of an issue. For months I have operated a stand-up forklift, but I just told the company that I can't do that anymore. I just can't take the pain. I don't know if using the forklift caused the problem, but I do know it makes the pain worse. It feels like it is just going to rip apart, it's that tight."

Demonstrating where he felt the pain, B pointed to the anterior thigh, from the trochanter to the knee.

"Does it ever go below the knee?" I inquired.

"No, I don't think it ever does. It just hurts from here to here," he said, gesturing from his hip to the knee.

This is the moment in seeing clients that I have always relished. With a few details, it is hard not to let the mind jump to conclusions or make decisions about the possible causes. It is both an opportunity and a potential pitfall.

Listening to him, my first concept was meralgia paresthetica. It is often seen in workers, especially ones who have to wear a tool belt that may insult the nerve. The symptoms fit perfectly; pain that comes from near the ASIS and goes down the front of the thigh but not below the knee. I felt a little twinge of excitement as I had not seen a case of meralgia paresthetica in many months.

"Do you often wear a belt?" I asked, looking to confirm my suspicions.

"I always wear a belt," he said, pointing to the belt looped through his jeans. (Ask a poorly worded question and get an answer that is unhelpful.)

"No, I mean a tool belt at work. Something heavy that you have to wear around your waist," I clarified.

"Nope, never do," he replied.

Uh-oh. This suddenly makes the meralgia paresthetica idea a little less likely. It serves me right for jumping on the bandwagon just a little too soon. What I know after all these years is to think about *all* the possible reasons that would explain a symptom before leaning in any one direction.

With B, what would explain pain down the front of the leg? The list of possibilities I created in my head included:

- A neural issue from L3 or L4
- Referred pain from the gluteus minimus
- A local issue of the vastus lateralis
- An SI joint problem
- Meralgia paresthetica (still had to keep it on the list)

Given this list of possibilities, it was time to have B move to the table and check this out.

"Let's explore the tissue and see what I can find. That will help me determine the possible cause for your pain and what we might do about it," I stated.

B just looked at me with a look that was somewhere between clueless and fearful. This big guy suddenly looked like a fourth-grader being asked to come to the front of the class.

"Um, I've never done anything like this," he admitted. "I, uh, am not sure how this works."

Massive blunder on my part. Having done this for forty-plus years, I make assumptions that clients have ideas about what to expect. Worse yet, my own approach is very different than what they might think of as massage therapy. I need to walk them through the process and explain what and why. Explaining things thoroughly takes away the unknown (the unknown creates fear).

I remember seeing some research years ago regarding new patients in a health care setting. In that survey, it was discovered that new patients want the answers to four questions:

1. What do you think is wrong?
2. What are you going to do?
3. Is there anything I should or should not do?

4. How long will this process take?

Even if the new client does not ask these questions, they are still thinking about them. Great clinicians answer them anyway. It was my time to correct my mistake and redirect the session in a way that resonated with B.

"What I am thinking about are four or five reasons that might explain your leg pain. I could make a case for all of them, but I need to explore this further to know which one is the most likely. One of the ways I explore this is simply to use my hands to examine your muscles, looking for restrictions, tenderness, and especially anything that recreates the symptoms. If I press on an area and it is related to your leg pain, you will know immediately. Your feedback is really important to this process. To do that, I am going to ask you to remove your shoes and your jeans and then lie on the massage table. You can leave on your shirt, everything we will treat will be from the low back down. I should have a better idea of what is going on after we finish. Then, I can tell you not only what I think is causing your pain, but what you might do or avoid doing. I will also have a better idea about how many sessions might be necessary. Sound like a plan?"

"I'm in," he said, almost jumping on the table. "how do you want me?"

What a difference a little time explaining the process makes! B was now excited, not tentative.

"Do you ever have low back pain?" I inquired, before beginning the treatment.

"Nope. I feel really lucky as I know a lot of people who really struggle with back pain. I can't ever remember hurting there."

His answer made the possibility that this leg pain is a nerve root issue much less likely. I could still explore this, but I moved to the end of the list.

This is another moment in a session that is always a landmark for me. Where does one place their hands to begin? Where? Why? How?

If B is hurting in his leg, I am going to start right where he is feeling pain. Since I also wondered about a superficial nerve issue, I decided to begin with a more fascial approach, moving the superficial fascia in a transverse direction over the deeper fascia. To my surprise, the fascial movement was far better than I expected. To my dismay, I also could see some doubt in B's face.

"It seems like you are dancing around the issue," he said, not in a critical way but one of observation. "It feels like the pain is deeper than that."

Point made, point heard. My palpation told me that the fascia was moving well, he is telling me the problem isn't where I was. The little problem is that one of my approaches is to, as immediately as possible, go right to the pain, demonstrating to the person the relevance (and accuracy) of what I am doing. My experience is that it draws clients in, creating a sense of the power of the work. I just missed the target with B.

Changing strategies, I altered the angle of my hands to address the vastus lateralis more directly (a perpendicular angle to the muscle). As I felt clear restrictions in the tissue, I could see B react.

"Whoa. Is that tender!" he exclaimed. "I had no idea it hurt so much. Do you feel that?" he asked, looking for validation.

"Do you mean this little area here?" I replied, pressing into the restriction.

"Geez. What the heck is that?" B asked, as I let up on the pressure.

"That sir, is an area of a muscle called the vastus lateralis, a very big muscle in your thigh. One small area of this big muscle is restricted and very sensitive. (This wasn't exactly news to B.) I am going to slowly, but thoroughly, try to work this out. My hope is to keep the discomfort level at a point where it just feels good to you to have someone finally address what you have been feeling all along. If you find yourself recoiling from the pressure, I need to let up. It should just feel great to have me there, even if it is painful."

"You mean like a good pain, right? Even though it hurts, in a weird way it also feels so good to get in there. I knew there was a problem and boy, does it ever feel like the leg is the problem."

"Possibly," I replied.

"What do you mean?" B asked. "It certainly feels like right where you are is the center of it all."

"Maybe. But one possibility to consider is that there might be some other area that is also stirring up the muscle in your leg. Is the leg the real problem, or is there somewhere else that is setting it off? We need to keep that possibility in mind. Let's do some work with the leg first, then explore other areas."

This is another moment in the session that could go two different ways. In many other, if not most cases, I would have left the leg and explored other possible causes immediately. Why? Using the tenderness in the leg as a reference point, treating a distal area would allow me to return to the leg to reassess the tenderness. If treating the gluteus minimus or the SI joint would substantially reduce the sensitivity at the vastus lateralis, the relationship of one to the other would be very clear, to both myself and to B. Because B was so thrilled to have me pressing on the exact area where he senses is the source of his pain, I decided not to move to distal referring areas. That decision was also in response to my initially choosing the wrong strategy. Now that B is hyper-connected to what I am exploring, I don't want to move to another area, especially if I am wrong in that choice. Being off the track twice will not increase his confidence in me or the approach. It is best to take the more certain road at this point.

After spending enough time at his vastus lateralis, it was clear that B also needed a break from the intensity of what we just did. My sense is that we ended at just the right time. Enough work that he felt I was thorough, but not so much as to be overwhelming. Knowing when to stop is just as difficult as knowing where to begin.

"I am curious about something else. May I explore two other places that may play a role in your leg pain?" I asked.

While B was on his side, I explored the gluteus medius with slow and careful pressure. A few areas were tender, but nothing remarkable. Moving closer to the sacrum, I could sense him react.

"Tender?" I asked.

"I'll say," he responded. "What is really weird is that when you do that, I feel it in the middle of my leg, right where you just were. That is crazy."

"Not so crazy," I relayed. "This is what I was looking for -- an area in your hip that is connected to your leg pain. I think we found it."

The area that I was addressing was the long dorsal ligament. There is only minimal research data to support this idea, but in my clinical experience, it can refer pain to the vastus lateralis. At any rate, it did for B, and that is what matters. I also found his multifidi attachments at about S3 extremely sensitive; this point also had an echo effect into his thigh.

B was quiet for a minute, then I could sense he wanted to say something. I stopped what I was doing to pay full attention to whatever he needed to convey to me.

"I'm in man, all in. Whatever you need to do, whatever it takes, however much you need to do; I am all in. This is so great. You know, I have been to multiple doctors and no one has ever even touched my leg. This is awesome. I am so glad I did this."

Comments like this are wonderful, but I do not take them personally.

What is most remarkable is his transformation from skepticism to enthusiastic support for the efficacy of the work. How did that happen? It wasn't from some slick presentation with flip charts, there were no posters on the wall, no traditional client education. What convinced him was his own experience. If you want client buy-in, get results. Results matter. More than what you say, it is the experience you facilitate.

B's enthusiastic support of the work is also very likely to increase his chances of success as well. While the research shows belief in the efficacy of the approach to be crucial to success, I want to make one very clear distinction between B's attitude and the placebo effect. I have seen hundreds of clients like B in my career and many, if not most of them, required multiple sessions to attain results. I can think of scores of clients who had little to no improvement in the first four or five sessions; progress did not happen until the sixth session or later. If you know anything about the placebo effect, this is not how placebos work. Placebos are about instant results, not results gained very slowly over time. The principle that can really help B is not placebo, but some deep internal knowing that this approach may indeed be the answer. He didn't get that from me convincing him with words, but from his own experience. In cases where results can take weeks to surface, that internal knowledge is enough to keep working at this until results blossom. That trust in the efficacy of the work should never be taken for granted. Ever.

Similar Symptoms- Different Reasons

The premise of this book is that every client who graces our treatment room has a story to tell and is an opportunity for learning. Each client deepens our understanding of various aspects and principles of massage therapy, which then can be applied to future clients. On this particular day in my clinic, my first three clients embodied a principle question that anyone who does soft-tissue therapy should ask him/herself.

Glancing at my schedule on this particular morning, I was amused to find that my first three clients presented with hip pain, and all of them were returning for their second visit. This was not planned, but the contrasts and similarities were instructional.

I had asked all three men to see their physician to get a radiograph of the hip. In each of these three cases, the symptoms could possibly be the result of severe arthritic changes in the hip. It was better to rule out that possibility first. Luckily, each had access to their physician, who also thought getting an image was a good idea. Just to review, the classic symptoms of severe hip arthritis are a limited range of motion in all planes of motion, pain in the groin, and pain during extended walking.

Let's review each of their sessions individually.

Client #1: T

At his first session, T relayed the incredible onset of his hip pain.

"I was terrified, but somehow I knew I would figure a way out of this terrible predicament. I was in the garage working on my car when it suddenly slipped forward and pinned me against the wall. Nothing I could do would release my leg and no one could see me because the garage door was closed. I couldn't reach my cell phone to call for help and my wife wasn't expected home for hours. Miraculously, after about an hour, the garage door went up as my wife returned home unexpectedly. I don't know if I have ever been so happy to see her."

"Did your hip hurt immediately?" I asked.

"No, that's the thing. Most of the pain was in the lower left leg where it was pinned against the wall. The right hip didn't start acting up until months later. I don't understand that. If the accident was the cause, why didn't the hip start hurting right away? It's possible that the accident doesn't have anything to do with my hip pain, but I really think it does. It really hurts here," he said, pointing to his groin and lateral hip area medial to the rectus femoris, just distal to the inguinal ligament.

"If I walk any distance, it really hurts, especially if I am on an uneven surface, such as walking in the woods behind my home. Occasionally, I need to present my products at sales conventions and being on my feet for hours is very painful. The pain has a deep and aching quality and is always present at some low level, spiking with episodes of higher activity. The pain is better when I sit, but getting up from a seated position can be really difficult."

When I had measured his hip range of motion, it was limited in extension and internal rotation, but only moderately limited in external rotation. He had only a slight discomfort with hip flexion.

Session #2

"How goes it?" I asked. "Were you able to get the X-ray?"

"I was," he replied. "I brought a copy of the report for you to see, but the doctor said it looks pretty good. The only thing he saw was a little decrease in the joint space, but otherwise normal. That's good news, right?"

"That's very good news," I responded. "Now we just have to figure out what is causing your pain. Did you notice any improvement after our last session?" I asked.

"I did. I think all of it was really helpful, but that last thing you did was probably the most helpful of all."

What T was referring to was the work we did on the psoas and the iliacus at the end of the first session. In many ways, it makes perfect sense given his symptoms. Restrictions in the psoas will cause a loss of hip extension and quite possibly a loss of internal rotation of the femur. All of these were true for T. More telling, sitting was a relief; spending hours on his feet (where the psoas is at full length) created pain.

In his second and third sessions, my focus was primarily on the psoas and the iliacus. I treated the lesser trochanter attachment primarily when T was prone, as this approach was far more effective for his body type. I treated his iliacus both seated and prone. Side-lying and supine approaches for his iliacus were inefficient and uncomfortable for T.

How these muscles were affected by his trauma is a mystery to me (and to

T). He didn't even remember all the crazy Cirque du Soleil-like positions he attempted while trying to free himself from the car. When you think you might die alone in the garage, you do crazy things. The body pays a price, but at least he is alive to have those problems. (And he is a little more cautious when working on his car now!)

Client #2: M

I had seen M for his first session about three weeks ago. He presented with similar symptoms to T, mostly centered in the front of the right thigh and groin area. There was no specific incident that M could recall that precipitated this pain. It just slowly appeared over time, making his life increasingly difficult. Any spike in activity would almost immediately increase his pain; if the activity was too intense, he would also experience lower back pain. Extended periods of walking and mowing the yard exacerbated his symptoms. His backyard is very uneven, with a rather steep incline on either side. His symptoms are far worse when pushing the mower up the hill than when coming down.

When I checked his femoral range of motion, there was a noticeable restriction in internal rotation and hip extension, with only a slight limitation in external rotation. Since he had an appointment with his doctor already scheduled, getting an X-ray seemed like a reasonable approach.

The report from the radiologist was unremarkable. I had suspected that this might be the case as he was not clearly restricted in all planes, but M really wanted an X-ray to confirm this. Getting the all-clear, it was time to go to work.

When M happened to be prone, I brought his right foot off the table, as to move the foot to the buttocks (knee flexion). Almost immediately, his right buttocks raised off the table. I don't think M even realized what he was doing, but the implication was clear.

"Does this movement hurt you?" I inquired, thinking there may be a possibility he is splinting due to knee pain or something similar.

"What movement?" he replied. (That was all the answer I needed.)

The motion of his right hip (which is called Ely's test) indicates shortness of the rectus femoris muscle. To negate the stretch from below, the person rotates their hip, shortening the rectus femoris by moving the upper attachment downwards, pivoting the hip.

The emphasis of this second session was mostly on the rectus femoris, approaching it from multiple positions and in multiple length-tension positions. Work on the rectus was alternated with work on the multifidi to address his lower back discomfort.

Client #3: D

D's hip symptoms were quite similar to the other two men. Like T and M, sitting was generally fine, but any extended activity created groin pain. Like M before him, there was no specific incident that he could say initiated this pain. The major difference in D was that his range of motion was limited in all planes of motion. We had done some very general work in the first session, and he was returning for a follow-up session.

"I have something I need to show you," was his opening remark. (That is seldom a good thing.)

Handing me the report, the verdict was in, and it wasn't good. Severe arthritic changes in the joint (as I had suspected). The look of worry on D's face said it all.

"I can't have surgery now, I just can't. I know the doctor thinks we should, but the timing just can't work right now. My wife needs me too much," said D, with such sadness in his eyes.

Stillness pervaded the room. I had remembered D telling me about his wife's very strange health problem, an odyssey that no physician seemed yet to solve. From the hospital to a rehab center, D was right there by her side. Being out of commission, even for a little while, was out of the question.

I broke the silence with a question.

"After our last session, did you notice any difference?"

"I did," D replied. "I don't know if I moved better, but I must have been better because I didn't think about my hip very much. Plus, my back was definitely better. That I noticed when getting in and out of the car and helping my wife when she was trying to walk."

"Okay, then I have a plan," I asserted. "It's not like you have to have this replacement immediately, but it is probably inevitable. Check with your doctor, I'm sure he will agree it is not time-sensitive. On the other hand, the danger is that if your hip has limited range, your low back will compensate.

I think we can treat the muscles around your hip to help you be more comfortable, while also addressing the muscles of your back to prevent them from getting over-worked. That should buy us enough time. Sound like a plan?"

D enthusiastically agreed, and this is the plan we enacted. I saw him every three weeks until he was able to get the replacement, which went flawlessly.

Three successive clients, all with hip pain in approximately the same location, and three very different reasons for the same symptom. (And people wonder if I ever get bored doing bodywork!)

The Wallpaper Wars

"Hi D, nice to see you," I said. "You can come on back."

"Okay, but you might have to help me," my client replied, struggling to rise from the chair.

"What the heck," I exclaimed. "What in the world happened?"

After helping her to my treatment room, she began to relay the whole story.

"My son just purchased his first home and I volunteered to help him remodel, starting with removing some very old wallpaper. We had rented a steamer, but even that didn't help get that old wallpaper off the walls. I wonder if the previous owner used superglue or something to fix the paper to the wall. Mostly, I had to use muscle power to pull it off the wall. Not long after we were done, which seemed like it took forever, I started to have this deep aching pain in my hip, which kept getting worse as the night went on."

"Where do you feel the pain is centered? Did the pain come on suddenly, or did it slowly develop afterward?" I inquired.

"The pain is really mysterious, unlike anything I have had before. Most of the pains I have had are easy to point to, but this is a deep ache that I cannot locate. I feel pain in the groin, but not in the way that a groin pull would feel. I feel a real tightness here (pointing to the pectineus area), but it isn't exactly painful when I press on it. At the same time, it hurts above my waist, all the way up in here (she pointed to the ASIS area), but again, it doesn't really hurt when I press on it. How weird is that? I thought I was being so careful! I even sat down most of the time and didn't do any of the high work above my head."

"Could you describe the motion of removing the wallpaper? I want to visualize your exact motions," I instructed.

"I was only doing the lower part of the wall and this part of the wallpaper seemed to be the most cemented on the drywall. To avoid hurting my back, I sat on a low stool pretty much the whole time. I was grabbing the wallpaper at about shoulder height and pulling downward to the floor. It was slow going the whole time, but I worked for hours. Not long after returning home, the pain began. I couldn't lift my leg; getting up from a chair was almost impossible. My husband had to help me in the bathroom, and I slept in a recliner because lying on the bed was impossible. I barely slept. Now, I can hardly stand up, but once up, I can slowly adjust to the position. Moving my leg forward while walking is very painful."

Helping her on to my table, I mentally ran through some potential possible causes.

My first thought was to lift her leg to create passive hip flexion. As I did this, she winced in pain. If passive movement created pain, that could indicate a much more serious intra-joint pathology. Why would that be, coming on so quickly without an abrupt trauma?

Or . . .

"Completely relax and allow me to lift your leg. I will go very slowly, and we can do it several times if you'd like."

It took her several times to allow me the full weight of her leg and to relax and let me lift it. Indeed, as she relaxed, the pain during passive hip flexion disappeared. This explains why it was painful the first time I lifted her leg. In all likelihood, the muscles of the joint were hypersensitive to length changes and fired reflexively. This was defense, not defect. I did this movement at first with her knee straight, then with the knee flexed. The hip flexion movement was fine until somewhere around 90 degrees of hip flexion when she felt a pinching pain in her groin.

"Describe the position you were in again. You were sitting in a chair and forcefully pulling down and forward correct?" I asked, demonstrating this action to her.

"Yes, and most of the work was to my left, so I was leaning that way while I was pushing my right leg outward (abduction) a bit for stability."

At that moment, it was very clear to me which muscle took the brunt of the strain. I suspected that the muscle at fault was a hip flexor; the possible culprits were the psoas, iliacus, and tensor fascia latae. Unfortunately, I could not use resistive testing to differentiate them; when such irritation exists, every muscle will test positive. Of the aforementioned muscles, the iliacus was the perfect functional match, as it creates pelvis-on-femur flexion, where the psoas creates femur-on-pelvis flexion. Because D was sitting, she was forcibly creating pelvis-on-femur flexion for hours. This is not an action we do often, let alone doing it with force for hours on end. In addition, the iliacus, unlike the psoas, is very sensitive to abduction, which she was doing with her right leg to stabilize movement to the left.

After carefully treating the iliacus, D was surprised to discover that getting up from my treatment table was much easier than expected. She gingerly took a few steps, finding them less painful than before the treatment. I encouraged her to alternate sitting and standing often in the next day or so. The improvement was rapid indeed, with a relatively good sleep in her own bed on the first night. In about two days, the pain was completely gone. The wallpaper, alas, did not fare as well.

Two Roads Diverged; I Took Both

Her message sounded alarming: severe cramping, pain, and numbness in her arm/hand. Having seen her son for severe trigger finger work (which turned out very well), this person thought of calling me for help with her arm and hand pain.

When I met with C, she pointed to the back of her index finger and thumb on her right hand.

"I have been having terrible cramping and pain in this area for several days now. It comes on intermittently, and the discomfort is awful. I read on the web that massage might help, but it is so sensitive, I couldn't even think of massaging it right now."

"Where exactly do you feel it?" I asked, trying to get a clear sense of the possible causes.

"Right here," she said, pointing to the dorsal side of the thumb, index finger, and possibly the middle finger. "The cramping doesn't go above the wrist," she added.

"Is there anything that you know that might have caused this? Is there anything you can do to relieve it?"

"I can't think of any reason why this is happening. Bending my wrist back like this seems to relieve it if I keep it there for a while," she said, putting her wrist in extension.

I mentally reviewed the possible causes of pain in the dorsal aspect of the thumb. I could think of three right away: *De Quervain's* syndrome, radial nerve entrapment, and possibly a referral coming from the extensor carpi radialis muscles. Direct treatment of the local issue was clearly out of the question -- C was extremely apprehensive about letting me touch the area of pain. Directly addressing the area of symptom presentation isn't smart if it is highly sensitive. If you suspect there might be a snake in the bushes, kicking the bushes isn't the best way to find out.

"Are you sure that both the cramping and numbness are only on the back of your hand?" I asked, trying to clarify that this could be a radial nerve issue.

"I can't be sure. When it hurts, it just hurts, and I have to admit that I really do not know," she relayed with some embarrassment. This point was important, but now unclear. The radial nerve serves the back of the hand, while the median nerve serves the palmar side of the thumb and index finger.

Her description was not going to help me determine which nerve might be involved.

The fact that C demonstrated to me that wrist extension decreased her symptoms could indeed point to the radial nerve, as the nerve is slackened by extension of the wrist. However, this position also slackened the wrist extensors, making it hard to discern whether the nerve or the muscle was relieved by wrist extension.

"What if we stretch the wrist in the opposite position?" I said, starting to move her wrist into slight flexion.

C gave me a look of fear as though I'd asked her to run across a busy interstate. "On second thought, let's not do that."

I was now officially stuck. The tests to implicate muscle vs. nerve are provocative -- not a great choice when symptoms are so active.

Faced with two diverging roads -- one muscular and one neural -- I decided to take both. I would treat in a way that would alleviate nerve entrapment with no possibility of irritating it. On the muscular front, I would treat the extensor carpi muscles while being careful not to irritate the nerve by stretching it or putting pressure on the nerve itself. That meant not stretching the muscle or putting direct pressure anywhere near where the radial nerve is located.

I treated the triceps brachii first, as the radial nerve lies between the muscle and the bone. All the treatment was a lifting compression to avoid putting pressure on the nerve. The supinator was next, using pressure with no stretch and carefully avoiding the area where the radial nerve might be. I performed a fascial release, stopping before I approached the area of symptoms near the wrist.

On the muscular side, I treated the extensor carpi muscles with careful slow friction in the direction of the muscle fibers. I did this with the wrist in flexion to keep the radial nerve in a slackened position.

C's symptoms were much improved by the third half-hour session. It became clear that the problem wasn't the radial nerve after all; it was the extensor carpi radialis brevis.

The idea that a therapist can precisely narrow down the cause of pain in one session is just that -- a wonderful idea. In reality, solving problems is a messy business. It isn't always clear which path to take. When you aren't positive, just make sure that choosing one possibility doesn't aggravate another suspected cause. When the roads diverge (and if it is possible), take both.

Chapter Five: Not Magic, Anatomy

Central Sensitization and the Master Volume Control

Accompanied by her mother, my newest client, a young woman of 14 years, carefully described her symptoms.

"This pain began several months ago, actually more a deep ache than a pain. It was gentle at first, then increased over time, starting first in my calves and then it spread to my ankles."

"Was it more one side than the other?" I inquired.

"It started on the left but quickly spread to the right as well. The pain has kept me from doing many of my favorite activities. Now, my knees hurt, and I cannot play soccer, basketball, or any serious athletic activity. In fact, just going for a walk is hard. The longer this goes on, the more limited I am."

I informed D that, using my hands, I wanted to explore the musculature of her legs. The moment I pressed on her tibialis anterior, she recoiled in obvious discomfort. Pressure on the posterior calf created the same reaction, as did any pressure near the ankle. Sensing that further palpation in this area was unwise, I decided to go elsewhere.

I cautiously palpated the rectus femoris about mid-thigh and again D recoiled, but slightly less than when I palpated her lower leg. With so much widespread pain, I began to think about other possible mechanisms and explanations. Turning to her mother, I asked whether they had consulted a physician.

"That is part of what makes this situation so perplexing," stated her mother. "My daughter does not seem to fit in any of the traditional boxes and no one seems to want to pursue treating her pain because it isn't life-threatening. It is, however, life-altering. We are at wits' end."

The mother went on to describe the many health-care disciplines they had tried. On the good news side, all of the medical conditions that I would be concerned about were already explored. With these eliminated, I could explore the soft tissue possibilities safely, as other providers eliminated some of the maladies that could create her widespread symptoms.

As I had been speaking to the mother for perhaps five minutes, I happened to notice that D, while lying on my table, had been applying pressure to her throat the whole time. Her mother, being aware that I was noticing her daughter's rather peculiar action, felt compelled to explain.

"My daughter often applies pressure to the front of her neck. Whenever there is a moment, especially when she lies down, she presses her throat."

D looked rather embarrassed at having this revealed to me, but she did not take her hand off her throat.

"Generally, we do what we do for a reason," I assured her. "There must be some reason you find pressing on your throat helpful."

"I don't know why," she admitted, "but pressing here seems to help me feel more relaxed," she said, gesturing to her throat. "It just quiets me."

"If I am gentle, may I explore the muscles in the front of your neck?" I asked. "Perhaps is a reason that pressing on them is helpful."

I began first with a mobility test of her hyoid bone and discovered that it did not move symmetrically. Movement to the left was restricted, implicating restriction in the omohyoid and digastric on the right. After releasing these two muscles, I retested the mobility, finding it much improved. I showed D how to move her own hyoid to relax and mobilize the muscles attached to it. This movement gave her both a measure of comfort and validation. The sternohyoid and sternothyroid were very sensitive bilaterally, as was the sternal head of the sternocleidomastoid. I showed D how to self-treat these muscles as well. This was important on several levels. Instead of telling her to stop pressing her throat, I showed her how to address it more effectively.

Returning to her quadriceps muscles, I replicated the exact pressure used earlier in the session and D did not react or recoil. Increasing my pressure, I was able to thoroughly explore and treat the quadriceps, locating and isolating selected areas of restriction, a far more normal reaction. I could see that D and her mother were astonished at how quickly the leg sensitivity had diminished after treating D's neck; an explanation was in order.

"The reason the neck treatment affected the lower body so dramatically has to do with central sensitization, an overexcitement of the central nervous system. You could think of the central nervous system as a master volume switch; if it is over-excited, everything below it will also be excited. Conversely, turn down the volume in the central nervous system, and everything below quiets down in response. Research has shown that certain areas of the body, such as your neck, can cause central sensitization much more quickly than other areas. By quieting a powerful source of input like your neck, the rest of your body also relaxed, making it possible for me to massage your legs more precisely. Pretty cool, huh?"

"Very cool!" chimed in D.

"That seems like magic," her mom exclaimed.

"Just the magic of our incredible nervous system," I responded.

Ferraris, Brakes, and Trills

Greeting S and her mom in my waiting room, I could see the worried look on both of their faces.

"My daughter is very serious about her music," the mom began. "She works very hard at it, and we are worried that this could be a real problem going forward."

"What instrument do you play?" I asked.

S's face immediately took on a look somewhere between pride and embarrassment.

"Four instruments, actually. The piano, string bass, the guitar, and the baritone horn."

"Let me guess. Is the problem in your left hand?" I inquired.

"It is," replied S with a little surprise in her voice.

"Am I correct in remembering that the baritone horn is held with the left hand and the valves are played with the right?"

"Yes, that's correct," S answered. "The pain I feel in my arm and hand started after a long session of playing the baritone. My school band played in the Fourth of July parade, which was unusually long this year. The pain started the next day."

"Show me where you hurt," I instructed.

S pointed to her flexor digitorum muscles on her left forearm.

"It is a deep ache and when it starts, I cannot continue playing."

"Did you notice any pain before the parade episode?" I asked.

"Not really," she answered. "One thing I did notice is that I wasn't able to do trills and more intricate passages in the last few weeks. It seemed like the more I practiced them, the worse I got. I also don't understand why it now hurts on this side of the arm (pointing to the extensors). When I press down on the keys or strings, doesn't it involve the muscles on this side (pointing to her flexor muscles) of the arm?"

"Correct, but it is a little more complicated than that," I replied. "Put your hand over my extensor muscles and feel what happens when I contract my finger flexors, like playing the guitar. Do you feel all that movement?"

"Wow, that's more movement than I thought," said S. "How come?"

"Two reasons," I replied. "First, every push with your finger requires these extensor muscles to lift the finger upwards to repeat the motion. That's the simple part. Second, and much more complicated, the extensor muscles control the descent of your finger to its intended target. When you press down the strings on the bass or guitar, do you always attack them with equal intensity?"

"No, she said. "Varying the pressure is how you get the differences in tone."

"Exactly", I concurred. "Nuances of pressure are made possible by the control of the extensor muscles, more than varying the power of contraction of the flexors. Whenever I think about this concept, I think of a chance meeting with someone who was parking his new Ferrari. I was totally awed by this amazing vehicle, especially since I had never actually seen one. Seeing my fixed stare at the imposing engine in the back of the car, he looked at me and declared that the engine is not the most impressive feature of the car. As I scanned the car with my eyes, I couldn't stop looking at the engine. Smiling patiently, he kept saying over and over that the engine isn't the most impressive feature. I knew he was guiding me to something, but I could not imagine what. After what seemed like an eternity, it hit me; it had to be the brakes. The owner smiled and offered that making a car go incredibly fast isn't terribly difficult, but stopping a car moving that fast requires an amazing feat of engineering.

"The same principle is true in your body. When one muscle contracts to make an action happen, the opposite muscle must control the quality and speed of that action. Like the big engine, the muscles creating the action get all the attention. The unsung heroes are the muscles controlling the action. In physiology, that function is called eccentric contraction, and it is one of the hardest jobs a muscle can do," I explained.

"Is that why I had a hard time doing trills?" S asked. "Was that an indication of when this problem began?"

"Great insight," I exclaimed. "It was probably the first sign of muscle fatigue and potential injury. Many of my athletic clients also notice little control failures before there is ever an obvious sign of pain. The more you learn to pay attention to smaller cues, the more likely you are to prevent more serious problems. Athletes and musicians both discover that the body is their real instrument, and massage therapy is a great way to further that self-discovery process."

"I never really thought of my music practice as athletics. Can you get me out of P.E. on Monday?" S quipped.

“Nice try,” said her mom with a smile. “Not happening.”

The Loudest Voice

"I think it might be worse," she said. "The problem might be spreading to other areas of my arm."

My eyes widened as I tried to make sense of what M was telling me. M was a pianist who had first come to see me six days ago with pain in her right lateral epicondyle. I had only seen her once, but three days after that treatment she sent me an email in which she was ecstatic at the results achieved. How could things have gone south just days since the email?

"Gosh, I am a little stunned," I admitted. "I thought your elbow was significantly improved after our session last week."

"Well, it was better, but now I am feeling the pain here," she stated, pointing to her triceps brachii muscle. "I don't think I ever felt pain here before. Perhaps the problem is more widespread than I thought."

"Before we began the work last week, you mentioned that the action of brushing your teeth was extremely painful. Were you able to brush your teeth with your right hand this week, or did you have to use your left hand again because of the pain?"

"Um, no. I have been brushing my teeth using my right hand for probably the last four days," she stated, giving me a puzzled look. "I kind of forgot how difficult that was for me."

"Are you still taking as much medication for pain as you were before we worked last week?" I asked.

"No, I haven't taken anything for the last few days," she admitted.

"That's good," I said. "But, I am still a little confused as to how you see the problem as worse since two of the markers for improvement, teeth brushing and medication use, are significantly better."

"I guess I am just concerned about this new area of my arm surfacing now," M admitted.

"May I ask how you would rate the pain and, maybe more importantly, how much this new area of discomfort affects your daily life?"

"This pain seems to have a different quality than the one I first came in with. While the original pain was debilitating, this pain is a sensation of fatigue and a deep ache. As a pianist, I have also been practicing a lot more this week, getting ready to perform a new piece."

"Who was the composer?" I inquired.

"It is a piece by Franz Liszt," she responded.

(If you are at all familiar with the piano literature, compositions by Liszt are massive works and physiologically challenging to play. Liszt had large hands and virtuoso technique; his pieces are often incredibly fast, powerful and extremely demanding.) M demonstrated for me some of the difficult passages via "air piano" -- the large chords and powerful pounding on the keys involved used lots of forceful elbow extension.

"May I tell you a story about one of my clients before we continue?" I asked. "I think you might find it helpful. I had seen this woman many times over the last few months; she had several very painful muscular issues due to a car accident. When I asked her how she was doing at her appointment last week, she complained of pain in her big toe. I probably gave her a look of confusion and concern. She, however, smiled and told me how delighted she was to have toe pain. Her point was that she, for many years, has had low grade pain in her big toe. After her car accident, multiple other areas of the body were of much greater concern to her nervous system. The toe pain was pushed far down the pain hierarchy. As she said, 'In the world of pain, the loudest voice wins. If I am aware of my toe aching, I know I must be getter better.' I think she nailed it. Do you see how that translates to your own experience?"

"I think I do," she replied. "The intense elbow pain overshadowed anything coming from the triceps, which now has the louder voice. Turning down the volume of the original pain allowed me to hear messages coming from the triceps."

"Absolutely," I agreed. "The triceps discomfort was likely there before, but the Liszt composition places an extreme demand on a muscle that was already somewhat compromised. The confluence of both factors is probably the reason it is speaking rather loudly to you right now."

"That makes a lot of sense," M replied. "After you treat it today, I think there are two things that I can do to help. First, I'll change my practice routine to limit the stress on that area. I got the message; the triceps doesn't need to yell to get my attention anymore."

"And second?" I asked.

"I am going to ask my triceps to use an inside voice!" she replied.

What Is Happening to Me?

"I'm scared. Am I having a stroke or something?"

These are not the kind of things one wants to hear in a continuing education seminar. As I looked over at her corner of the room, I could see several therapists gathering around her. Whatever was happening wasn't good.

As I approached, I could see that Ms. A was shaking rather uncontrollably, a kind of deep shiver that went through her whole body. The other students looked on with both concern and fascination. They glanced at me with that "You know what you are doing, right?" look.

Let me back up just a bit. In our training, we were just doing some very specific treatment on the quadratus lumborum muscle. Ms. A had had some back issues for quite a while, but she had assumed it was a more serious problem than a muscular issue, one that she had neither the time nor money to pursue. As her partner therapist was zeroing in on the exact spot of discomfort, she involuntarily flinched against an exquisitely sensitive spot. That is when all hell broke loose. Ms. A began to feel very cold and her body shook uncontrollably. Her partner really became concerned when Ms. A stated that her face was going numb.

It is one thing to have an unexpectedly powerful reaction to bodywork in the quiet of a massage room; it is another thing to have one with an audience. The fear in the room was palpable and not helpful. As therapists began to gather around, I politely asked them to vacate the room so that I could attend to Ms. A completely and without distraction. Reluctantly, they complied.

Putting blankets on Ms. A, I encouraged her to tell me what she was feeling, but I also kept reminding her of the present circumstances. Whatever this reaction was, it was important that she orient herself to the present moment. She described the neural storm that was going through her body as though she was witnessing it. As much as possible, we just kept observing her experience, without getting too lost in the fear of what it might mean. Most remarkably, she could watch the whole process as it happened to her. She did feel a bit out of control, yet she wasn't terribly afraid.

The entire episode lasted about fifteen minutes. Afterward, the feeling in her face and body returned to a more normal state, but she was exhausted. Since she lived close by and this was near lunchtime, she decided to go home and rest before returning to the seminar.

After the "storm", my class had lots of questions, as one might expect. The obvious one is "What just happened here?"

There are times when bodywork can bring up a very emotional experience, perhaps even bringing up a traumatic memory long forgotten. Ms. A had no such memory or emotion connected to her experience. Generally, this experience was far more physical than emotional. While addressed in the literature, very little is known about referrals to the autonomic nervous system. Autonomic reactions such as sudden goose-bumps, lacrimation, or feelings of coldness aren't common in clinical experience, but they do happen. This is not an easy area to research, but there are studies that give us insight into autonomic effects. I see autonomic effects only a few times a year, but the experience of the client is always one of surprise and bewilderment. Again, the experience of the client is very different than what they experience with a spontaneous emotional release.

The next morning in class was quite remarkable. Therapists in the seminar who knew Ms. A knew all too well that she was decidedly *not* a morning person. She was typically dragging and not a happy camper until noon. On this morning, Ms. A came early to class and was animated and full of energy. Her friends just looked at her like she was on drugs or something. Finally, one of them commented on her energy level and attitude.

Ms. A responded by describing how well she slept and that she awakened early, before her alarm. Her friends were stunned. They just kept looking at her like she been replaced by someone who looked exactly like her.

When Ms. A had no explanation for her high energy level, one of her friends asked her if she thought it had anything to do with the experience she had the previous day. I find it absolutely remarkable that Ms. A's reaction revealed that that thought never entered her mind. While obvious to everyone else in the room that these experiences might be connected, Ms. A never gave her powerful experience another thought after it was all over. All she knew was that she felt great.

Why would she have so much more energy? She did present like a different person. Research insights do give us some possible explanations and they are absolutely fascinating.

For the recipient, it feels like the offending exquisitely tender point is only tender when being pressed upon. (Have you ever heard comments like, "I was fine until you started poking around?") The research data reveals that those points are always sending low-level impulses to the central nervous system. This phenomenon is called "spontaneous electrical noise". Your nervous system does not do well when it is being bombarded with extraneous input. That's why we like quiet when trying to concentrate. It is also why calming the body is calming the mind.

This is an extremely important point. There is a class of medications called benzodiazepines, which are commonly prescribed when a patient has muscle spasms. Interestingly, these same medications are also prescribed for people with anxiety. Calm the body, calm the mind. One affects the other.

When the therapist happened, albeit a bit by accident, on the significant spot in Ms. A's back, it released a torrent of input into her Central Nervous System (CNS). What Ms. A did not know is that, in all likelihood, that spot was constantly bombarding her central nervous system with extraneous stimuli. When her therapist stepped on the proverbial "landmine" and the input spiked and then plummeted, the input into her CNS abated as well. When the CNS functions better, everything is better, including sleep, cognition, and emotional health. While the process was anything but comfortable for Ms. A and not an outcome that should ever be intended (creating a crisis), the long-term outcome for Ms. A was excellent. It was a very instructive experience for all of us.

Chapter Six: Turning the Tables

"Nothing builds confidence like

lack of knowledge."

Feedback, Albeit Humbling

It was a Saturday and I was home in Champaign, IL. If I am home, the odds are that I will also be at the clinic, trying to see all the clients I need to get into my crazy schedule. This particular Saturday was no different.

Perhaps some of you find yourself doing this, but I tend to find myself running in themes. Whatever research I am reading sparks an interest that colors what I see and experience. At this particular time period, I was preparing for Colloquium 2016, which was entitled The Path to Mastery. One of the areas that I was researching was client communication and its relationship to creating results.

The research I was reading came from the field of psychotherapy, a field that has many parallels to the field of massage therapy. I seem to learn more when reading studies of fields outside my own, perhaps because I know and acknowledge my lack of training in the field and it helps me be more open to deeper insights. In any case, the research on feedback was fascinating. In this particular study, the researchers were comparing informal feedback solicitation with more formal feedback collection. For an informal basis, the therapist would simply verbally check in with the client at least twice during the session. This was being compared with more formal feedback in the form of a written card handed to the client in the middle of the session and at the end.

Ultimately, the research study was scrapped. Why? When they analyzed the video (all the sessions were recorded), hardly any of the therapists who were supposed to solicit feedback informally actually did so. The researchers could not compare the formal to the informal because there was no informal feedback collected.

Before you think to yourself, "I always ask for feedback," I'd just like to point out that all of these therapists knew they were in a research study comparing two forms of feedback. More importantly, they knew the sessions were being videotaped. And still, they did not solicit feedback. The therapists insisted they did so, until they were shown the video of the sessions.

Additional research showed that an increase in feedback collection resulted in some incredibly impressive gains in clinical outcomes. It is such a simple act, but simple and easy are not the same thing. It takes courage to ask. It takes skill to change course.

Ever since reading these studies, I made it a personal mission to make absolutely sure I ask my clients for feedback, doing so at least twice during a session. I must also admit I almost never ask for feedback after a session is over. In a way, what is the point? It's too late to do anything then.

On this particular Saturday, I answered the phone after my last client of the day had just left. The woman on the line had neck pain and wanted in on that same afternoon. None of the therapists in my clinic had time to see her, so I decided to extend the day and see her immediately.

This is slightly embarrassing, but clients who come to my office know that I am very hard to get to see, for a multitude of reasons. Not surprisingly, this client was thrilled to get to see me personally and on such short notice.

Sitting down with her, she reviewed her neck pain and the circumstances surrounding it. I'd share those details with you, the reader, but they are unimportant. What is important is that ten minutes into the session, after very thorough and precise work on several muscles on the right side of her neck, I stopped the session to practice what I preach.

"I just wanted to check in with you. Does the approach I am using feel like it is effectively addressing your neck pain? Does what I am doing feel relevant to your pain? Would you like me to alter what I am doing to be more effective?" I asked, thinking about the aforementioned articles I had read the night before.

Looking up at me, she gave me her response.

"You know the pain is on the other side, right?"

Holy crap! Are you kidding me? How horrifying. (Lucky her that she got to see me.) As embarrassing as her answer was, it is also unpleasant to ponder how long this blunder would have continued before it was corrected. When would she have said something? Would she just think I had some grand plan, or would she just think I'm a completely over-rated idiot?

This was a humbling experience. Yes, we can all make serious mistakes. It is not possible to fix a problem of which you are unaware. Feedback makes course correction possible.

Just for the record, I did spend extra time with her (making up for the time I was off in the Netherlands). I made darn sure that she did not leave my office until significant progress was attained regarding her neck pain. She left happy, I left humbled. Such is life in the clinic.

Role Reversal

I was tired. Really tired. The kind of tired that my mom used to call "bone-tired." Seeing an opening in one of my massage therapists' schedule, I jumped at the chance to get some work done.

Jennifer walked me back to her treatment room and asked what my goals for the session were for this evening.

"First, I am exhausted. Too much travel, and then I have seen a lot of clients from the moment I stepped off the plane."

"Any specific areas bothering you?" she inquired.

"Yes, my neck has been an issue for the past several days."

"Where specifically?" she asked. "Is it pain or lack of range?"

"Well, umm, it, uh. . ."

"You've got to be kidding me," I thought to myself. Talk about sounding inarticulate. I know my neck has been bothering me for days now, and yet, when asked, it sounds like I've checked my brains at the door.

Thinking more about this and moving my neck, it became clearer to me what specifically was happening. "It is worse when I turn to the right," I replied. "I seem to have pretty good range to the left but turning to the right is restricted."

"When you turn to the right, do you feel it on the right side of your neck or on the left?" she asked.

Again, I had to stop and think about this and do the movement again. Jennifer waited patiently for me to get a bit clearer, moving and taking an inventory of my neck. As I was taking this neck inventory, I was immediately transported back to my experience in a Japanese hotel in 1992.

I had just arrived in Japan that evening, the first night of a six-week Rotary scholarship to study the Japanese health care system. I was exhausted from the flight but discovered that the hotel had massage available. I was worried that I might not have the chance to get a massage in Japan again, so I did not want to squander this opportunity. Settling into my room, I called the front desk and ordered a massage. Due to my terrible Japanese language skills, I wasn't sure if I ordered massage, food, or laundry service. Luckily, a massage therapist, a very petite female therapist who I would guess was near retirement age, showed up about twenty minutes later. As she entered my tiny hotel room, I suddenly realized that I had no idea how this would work.

There was no massage table, no space I could see for the massage. She began politely explaining how this could work, none of which I could understand. Assuming she was asking me to disrobe, I began removing my suit and tie, and then shirt. The horrified look on her face told me I was doing something quite wrong, so I ended up standing there like a three-year-old with my arms outstretched as she prepared my clothing appropriately. How humbling. All I kept thinking was, "Is this how my clients feel?"

By the way, that therapist almost killed me. Okay, not really, but, oh my goodness, she was strong. One would think that the sounds of suffering I heard myself making would cross communication borders, but evidently not in this case!

I realized that Jennifer was looking at me, waiting for an answer about my neck.

"The right," I blurted out. "It hurts on the right when I turn to the right."

"Fine," she said confidently. "It could be one of three muscles, all of which are contralateral rotators. Since these muscles rotate the head to the opposite side, they must let go to allow you to turn to the same side. Why don't you lie face up on the table and let's find out which one of the three is the major culprit."

The clarity and confidence of her approach put me completely at ease. We had a clear goal, three possible threads to follow, and it was clear that she knew what she was doing and why.

Again, I was lost in thinking about this from the client perspective. The sense of relaxation and ease I felt in response to her questions was a visceral experience. I knew that she knew what she was doing and why she was doing it. It created a sense of confidence about what was to come. She was in complete control, and I felt that as being incredibly reassuring.

As she began exploring the musculature of my neck, it was like a guided tour of my own body. I felt like someone had a flashlight and was walking me through empty rooms in my house that I had forgotten to reopen after a long and cold winter. We were opening the doors to rooms forgotten, pulling the sheets off the furniture, and dusting off the tables. It was a marvelous experience.

Lying face down, she began to explore the musculature and movement capabilities of my thoracic spine. In the upper thoracic spine, she pressed on a transverse process and I immediately felt it all the way up into my neck. At some deep level of knowing that I cannot articulate, I knew that this was the source of my neck issues. Mentioning it to her, she calmly stated that this is the attachment of the semispinalis cervicis, the same muscle that was most tender when I was face up. Plus, it fit perfectly with the symptoms I described.

Exploring further, she found other ancillary spots that I experienced as tender but had a deep sense of them being important to address, but not relevant to my immediate symptoms. Somehow, my nervous system knew that these spots were "old" areas that were once problematic, but now have been relegated to the background. How many times have I heard clients say that? Furthermore, how does the nervous system sense that?

The purpose of these table lessons has always been that each session is an opportunity for learning and professional growth. Sometimes, the best way to learn is through role reversal, putting oneself in the position of the one being served.

Who Is Assessing Whom?

"You could certainly tell who was the most experienced," stated my client with certainty. "It was interesting to perceive the distinct differences in abilities and experience between the therapists."

I am sure my eyes widened a bit at her statement. I was immediately lost in thought, thinking about the impact and gravity of her statement. Allow me to explain the context.

Ms. J was a previous client participant in an advanced level course I was teaching. She had returned for a follow-up session after her initial participation. In these courses, six therapists and I see clients who have predefined specific issues. In almost all cases, I have never met the clients; my only contact with them is a phone interview, making reasonably sure their problem is relevant to our training. This makes the context of the session as real as possible. Many of these clients have never had massage therapy, and I have no idea where the direction of the session might go. As a group, we interview, create assessment strategies, and problem-solve our way to a viable strategy, which is then executed. In its simplest form, we gather information, interpret the meaning of that information, and then respond. If the response is positive and what we expect, we are on the correct path. If not, we redirect. This is the hallmark of great problem-solving, no matter what the discipline.

How do we gather information? In our field, there are three primary avenues. First, we ask questions. Voltaire stated that you can judge a person's intelligence by the quality of their questions. In medicine, it is often stated that 90% of diagnosis can be done with a detailed case history alone. In the field of massage therapy, asking pertinent questions can influence treatment outcomes immensely. Second, what we observe is an essential aspect of gathering information. We observe the client's posture, movement patterns, and body language. These observations are then combined with the case history for possible connections. Third, we palpate. What is the quality of the tissue? How does the tissue respond to intervention? From our first training in massage school to advanced approaches in the field, the value of accurate and thorough assessment is stressed as essential to producing desired outcomes.

That is what makes Ms. J's statement so powerful. Who is assessing whom? While we therapists are concentrating on our listening, observational, and palpatory skills, our clients are doing the same to us. The assessment highway has two lanes. When she stated her ability to discern differences in therapists, my brain flashed back to her session during the training. Let's take each of the three avenues of information gathering from her perspective.

Listening: I remember watching Ms. J as she listened to the questions from my group of therapists. Watching her micro and macro facial expressions, she was reacting to the question and to the questioner. If the question seemed irrelevant or too vague, her expression revealed the disconnect. Questions that surprised and intrigued her were revealed in her body language and showed a connection with the therapist who asked such an insightful question.

Observation: I paid close attention to Ms. J's reaction to the group; she was observing us (including myself) closely. In fact, following her comment about the varying level of experience and abilities between therapists in the group, she also commented on how fully engaged some therapists were. How is it that she determined full engagement? I thought back to watching her eyes while she was lying supine on the table while one therapist was treating her. She was glancing around the room, observing the other attending therapists, who were not presently treating her. If those therapists were distracted or not paying attention to what the treating therapist was doing, she registered that as lack of engagement.

Palpation: This aspect of her experience at the training was absolutely intriguing.

"How is it that you determined one therapist was more experienced or competent than another?" I had to ask.

"The quality of their touch," she replied. "Some therapists, from the initial contact, put their hands on me with complete authority; I felt a clarity about what they were feeling and why. It just put me at ease, like they knew what they were doing and were fully in charge. Other therapists seemed tentative, which might be a lack of confidence. The difference was quite noticeable."

I processed Ms. J's statements as we shared a moment of silence. So much of the focus of training in the field of massage therapy is centered around the therapist's assessment and subsequent response. Far less discussed is the reality that as we are assessing the people who grace our treatment table, they are assessing us as well. In our speech, in our body language, in our touch; what impressions are we giving them? Who is assessing whom?

Chapter Seven: Validation

"Touch is a form of communication.
Therefore, all the rules of good
communication apply to touch as well."

A Privilege and a Responsibility

Looking at my schedule on this morning, I happened to notice my first two clients were coming from quite a distance. One name I recognized, the other was a new client. Looking at my notes from the client I had seen previously, I familiarized myself with the session I had done for her about six months ago. The first client was the new person.

Sitting down with L, the new client, she began to recount her experience with pelvic pain that was truly life-altering. L shared that her pain began about three years ago after a surgery. Interestingly, L recounted the many ways that this pain had affected her life.

As L relayed her story, I was struggling to stay focused on the details because of the depth of her struggle and how gracefully she dealt with it. Two thoughts distracted me. First, it was hard not to wonder how I might deal with this kind of tragedy. Could I handle it with her grace and composure? One never knows. Second, it is humbling to acknowledge how a person I have never met can share such deeply personal stories. The trust and confidence she displayed is humbling and always inspires me to give my very best to people who are so open and honest. Do I unequivocally know I can help L? Absolutely not. But, I do know that I will do my absolute best to make a difference[MC5].

After L left, B was my next client. She, too, had presented with pelvic pain when she visited my office about six months previously. Before she described her present state, she reviewed her condition when we met earlier.

"I don't know if you remember, but I was in a terrible place when I last saw you. I seldom left the house, as the pain limited almost every activity I wanted to do. I was afraid to make any commitments, knowing that I would likely need to cancel because of the pain. I felt bad at work, because I never knew when I would feel well enough to keep going, which often made me feel guilty about shifting my tasks to someone else. Feeling bad about feeling bad made the problem worse. But, I couldn't help it."

"And now?" I inquired.

"I'm better, I'm really better," B stated.

"How do you know that?" I asked. It may seem like a strange question, but it is important to know by what criteria a client measures improvement.

"By what I can do," she answered. "I can work longer and be more active.

The other day, a co-worker asked if I could stay longer and I didn't hesitate. I only thought about it later, that a month or so I would never have said yes. I still have pain, but I know I must be better because I am doing more."

B's answer perfectly fit into the current understanding of pain science. For many years, providers have used a pain rating scale to assess the pain level of patients. (On a scale of one to ten, how much pain are you experiencing?) This scale is fraught with problems on multiple levels. What is a ten? Where is the reference point? The new Department of Defense and Veterans[MC6] Pain Rating Scale (DVPRS) is a wonderful response to that problem, as it also includes functional measures. A four on this pain scale is also accompanied with the following: This pain distracts me, but I can do usual activities. A seven means 'this pain is the focus of my attention and prevents me from doing my usual activities.' That is a much more understandable scale for everyone concerned.

While there are many possible causes to pelvic pain, both women had a similar, but unexpected muscular cause, the external oblique. In both cases, very careful and thorough treatment of the upper rib attachments made a world of difference in their experience of suprapubic pain. The most important areas addressed were at the rib attachments, not the muscle belly or the lower attachments.

Like L before her, B struggled with not only the pain she was experiencing, but also depression and hopelessness. Common to both was pelvic pain, something that couldn't be easy for either of them to seek help from a male massage therapist whom they did not know. Pelvic pain is very personal and very devastating. After seeking help and finding none from other health providers, these people often suffer in silence, telling no one about their plight. In that light, having a client present such problems is a distinct privilege and an honor. With that honor also comes great responsibility.

Validation

Walking the hallway to my waiting room, I was thinking about how much I enjoy seeing new clients. Each one is an unfolding story, both a mystery to be solved and also a lesson to be learned for both my client and myself; it is truly a collaborative experience. Walking into my waiting room, I was greeted by two vivacious women, a mother and daughter whose smiles lit up the room. Their delightful presence was all the more amazing given the sad story that was to follow.

Sitting in my office, the daughter, P, relayed to me the story of her painful odyssey over the last two years. P had been a fairly active person who radically changed her diet and exercise regimen during her second year of college in hopes to get in better shape. For about seven months she followed a strict schedule of running a few miles on a treadmill 6 to 7 times a week (with the treadmill set to a very high incline), supplemented only by stretching and an occasional hot yoga class.

After about eight months, she began to feel a build-up of knee pain on the underside of her patella. After noticing it for a few days, her knee pain went from annoying to excruciating. Since that day she had experienced constant knee discomfort and, at times, excruciating pain in the patellar region of both knees.

Her mother added to the history by listing all the health providers that her daughter had consulted with. The list was long and included primary care physicians, four different physical therapists, and several orthopedic doctors. On the good news side, there was nothing obvious in the X-ray findings or on any other test that had been conducted. She had been seeing a physical therapist for over a year, but the treatments (stretching and strengthening) hadn't made an appreciable difference.

"What an ordeal you have been through," I said, leaning back in my chair. "I'm sure it has been very difficult for both you and your parents as well."

"I just want you to know that I have proactively and religiously been following the physical therapy program. My physical therapist can vouch for my commitment, as I see her regularly and she continues to monitor my progress. A year later, I am still forced to make concessions in my daily life to accommodate for my knee injury, even recently having to break my lease in order to transfer to an apartment that is on the first floor."

Something about the tone of her voice struck me, as though at some point, her commitment and dedication to the therapy had been called into question.

"Has anyone done specific soft-tissue work on your legs?" I asked.

"The physical therapist has been doing stretching and strengthening," replied P.

"No, I mean focused massage strategies, where someone puts their hands on your muscles."

"She has done a little massage on my quads," replied P.

Not knowing what exactly "a little massage" means, I decided to start right in. Examining first the vastus lateralis, then the rectus femoris, I sank into the tissue with my fingers, moving very slowly and methodically with deep friction in the fiber direction of the muscle.

"Whoa," P said as I found an exquisitely sensitive area. "No one has done that before."

Moving the rectus femoris aside to address the vastus medialis, I could feel P's body react.

"I can feel that right under my patella," she said incredulously. "*That* is exactly the pain I feel under my kneecap."

"Perfect," I replied. "I am going to hold the pressure, as long as this is tolerable, until there is a substantial reduction in the pain at your knee. Tell me when that happens."

At one point I looked up to notice that P's eyes filled with tears. Starting to pull back, I was about to admonish her for not telling me the pressure was too much.

Sensing my reaction, she shook her head. "The pressure isn't too much," she shared. "This is so confirming. If you can press on my leg and recreate my knee pain, it means that my pain is real and that I am NOT making this up."

No kidding. Yes, the pain is real, as I can put my finger on it. Her statement also shed a light on her earlier statement about being dedicated to the prescribed treatment protocol. It is not uncommon, when patients do not improve, to have providers assume that the patient is not following the prescribed self-care. It is easier to question the patient's dedication than to question the accuracy of the diagnosis or the treatment regimen.

Sadly, P's statement is reflective of the experience of so many people who have suffered chronic pain. They often feel invalidated by both health care providers and, unfortunately, even family and friends. If no observable pathology can be seen on a diagnostic image, or if typical treatments don't work, the validity of the patient's experience is called into question.

Those of us in massage therapy should celebrate how confirming touch can be for our clients. Few other health professions can demonstrate such a direct relationship to the presenting symptom. If we can directly recreate the client's pain with our palpation, the relationship between the area being touched and the pain is rather obvious to everyone. No long explanations are necessary, no leap of faith is required. Whatever the beneficial physical mechanisms are, the emotional effect is just as powerful: worthy of being cherished and celebrated.

Three years later

I just saw P in my office, as she stopped by to see one of my staff for a maintenance session and to say goodbye. P graduated from college and, along with her whole family, is moving to a new city. She has resumed an amazing workout schedule and hasn't had the symptoms return in more than two years. Excited about her life, healthy and incredibly active, she is profoundly grateful for the help she received, and I am profoundly grateful to have played a role in her recovery.

This is Not Who I Am . . .

After greeting my new client L, we sat across from each other in an assigned area of my treatment space reserved for listening and learning. The beginning exchange with a new client is a profoundly special and often powerful experience; one that I cherish deeply. L recounted that her experience with pelvic pain began about three years ago after a supposedly routine surgery. Unfortunately, the pudendal nerve was traumatized during the procedure, and the symptoms began a month or two later. Her pain was an annoyance at first, then escalating gradually, increasing in both intensity and frequency. Workouts became more difficult and, as time progressed, even long walks provoked her symptoms. The longer the pain persisted, the more fatiguing it became for her. Like many people in pain, she also felt that this negatively affected her cognitive abilities; she noticed that her clarity of thinking and memory skills were much diminished. As L recounted the many ways that this pain had affected her life, her voice faltered, and a river of tears soon followed. After a long silence, she regrouped and made complete and forceful eye contact.

"I need to show you something," she said, pulling two pictures out of her purse. "This is me," she stated. "This," she said, waving her arm across her body, "is not who I am." While the tears began again, her eyes did not waver from direct eye contact with me. It was very clear that she didn't want me to simply glance at the photos, she wanted me to fully "get" what she was telling me.

The pictures were indeed stunning. Taken only a few years previously, the pictures revealed a woman who was fit, vivacious, and possessed an infectious smile. I would not have guessed that these pictures were of the same person sitting in front of me. L kept looking at me without saying a word, her eyes searching mine to see if I understood the gravity of what she was trying to communicate. I held my gaze on the pictures for a long time, sensing this is what she needed.

In this silence, my thoughts were lost in the reality of how chronic pain can devastate one's sense of self-identity. L's sense of herself is that vivacious person in the photos, which is why she carried these photos everywhere she went. Those photographs are a reminder that the person she is now is not who she believes herself to be. Sense of self is at the core of physical and emotional health, and this is an aspect of health upon which chronic pain can wreak great havoc. The dissonance between these two images of self, one present and one past, is the source of untold internal struggle and pain. It would be a different story if, over time, one stopped exercising and therefore gained weight. It is a very different thing when this happens *to* you, produced by circumstances out of your control.

I am sad to say that L, like many other people in chronic pain, did not have a great experience with the health care providers who were assigned to her care. Mostly, she felt invalidated by the way they related to her. Some were dismissive, some didn't listen, others just did not seem to care. Like that old saying, people don't care how much you know, they want to know how much you care. For people in chronic pain as well, it isn't just the symptoms they feel, it is largely about the impact of the pain on their perception of self. Until that is acknowledged, it is hard to progress. Like a GPS system, to get where you want to go, you also need to know where you are. Listening and acknowledging are the beginning steps of that path; the client must sense that you understand his/her current reality. Once that is established, real progress can happen. For L, she not only needed me to sense where she is now, but also where she came from. That's why the pictures were so important to her.

Pudendal nerve issues can be extremely complicated and difficult to treat. This nerve has three branches, the perineal nerve, inferior rectal, and the dorsal penile/clitoral. Much of the improvement we made was accomplished through very careful treatment to the piriformis muscle, the sacrotuberous ligament and Alcock's canal (the obturator fascia). My goal was to make movement more comfortable and to slowly increase her activity level. While those manual treatment protocols were taken, perhaps the most important action was to make sure that L felt "heard" and validated after our first appointment. Acknowledging her dignity as a person was the first step to healing.

After she left, I kept thinking about a quote from Ambroise Paré, a French barber-surgeon who lived in the 1500's.

> *"The ultimate duty of the physician is to cure*
> *occasionally, relieve often, console always."*

-Ambroise Paré (1510-1590)

This is timeless wisdom for all of us in health care.

Chapter Eight: Life Lessons

"You cannot change an outcome

until you deeply understand

the context that created it."

An Unforgettable Lesson

Some sessions and the lessons learned stay with you for a lifetime. Such is the case with B.

I have always enjoyed seeing B; she possesses the perfect combination of intelligence, insight, and compassion that makes her a very successful psychotherapist and a delight to be around. It is not surprising that she is such a successful therapist. On this particular day, she visited my office to address orofacial pain on the left side.

"Show me where you are feeling pain," I began.

B pointed to the left side of her face in a rather broad sweeping motion, so broad I couldn't really tell what she was pointing to. This made me wonder if she was unaware of the exact source or if the pain presentation was that diffuse. More questions left me still quite unclear, so I decided to move from verbal questioning to palpation. While she was seated, I examined her tissue for further clarification.

"How about this muscle?" I asked, pressing on her masseter.

"I think so," she said. Each area of the masseter seemed about equally sensitive, a bit unusual.

"And this?" I asked while exploring her temporalis.

"There too, I think," she answered.

Like the masseter, the temporalis was sensitive, but equally sensitive wherever I touched. Given the mass of the temporalis, that is a lot of territory to have the same sensitivity. A little alarm went off in my head, but I must admit I barely heard it. Why?

Given the presentation of her pain, both of these muscles were prime suspects. They both fit her symptom presentation. I wanted to put these muscles in the "treatment box." They seemed like perfect fits. First mistake.

If muscles have a problem, it is likely, but not a given, that they will have range of motion restrictions. I then measured B's interincisal opening with three successive readings, which were 41, 44, and 47 millimeters, respectively. For B's petite size, these readings were not indicative of notable restriction. In addition, the readings improved each time, something that our research endeavors have told us is a good sign. If the masseter and/or the temporalis are involved, why is the range of motion so unremarkable? Thinking about this more, I thought about other presentations where muscle length tests fine, but contraction reveals the problem. Range restriction is not the only sign of injury. If muscles have only one job, to contract, they will do that job less well in the presence of an injury.

"Do you have trouble with sustained chewing of foods, such as a bagel or a piece of steak? Do you find your jaw tired or painful afterward?"

"No, I can't say that I do. I chew gum occasionally and that never bothers me. I have never noticed the pain in my jaw or face being worse after chewing, but maybe I am just not paying enough attention to when it happens."

Somehow, deep inside, I found her answer to be unsatisfying. This was not the answer I was looking for. Perplexed, I had her lie supine on my table and proceeded to explore the orofacial musculature. When all else fails, it is back to palpation of the tissue in question.

I began with the fan-like temporalis, carefully palpating every millimeter. Starting first with the posterior section, I soon found some areas where the tissue felt restricted. It didn't take long.

"That's pretty tender," B remarked.

"Now we are onto something," I thought. "Do you feel it here too?" I asked, moving a few millimeters anteriorly.

"Yes, there too," she replied.

That process continued throughout most of the temporalis. I found many tender spots but none of them replicated her pain exactly. Again, at a deep level, I found this unsettling. Curious, I decided to explore the right temporalis for comparison. It too had many very sensitive areas, not much different than the left. If her pain is only on the left, why is there no substantial sensitivity difference between the left and right side?

I proceeded to explore the masseter on the left, starting first externally and then intraorally. As with the temporalis, I found numerous tender areas, none of which replicated her pain. The right masseter was just as tender as the left. I expanded the search to other orofacial muscles, each muscle having the same result. The alarm bells just got louder.

"What do you think?" B asked.

"I don't have the sense that we found the cause of your pain. I feel like I am missing something," I admitted. "Would you be willing to keep a little journal about this pain for me for a couple weeks? Writing down when you feel discomfort might pinpoint something for us that I am missing."

"Would you write that instruction down for me?" B asked.

B responded sheepishly to my quizzical glance. Writing down such a simple request seemed overkill, but I felt terrible seeing the embarrassment on her face.

"I know it seems strange," she admitted, looking very embarrassed. "I have been having so many senior moments lately that I do not trust myself anymore. Everyone thinks that they struggle with memory, but this seems far more serious. I often find myself in a room not knowing why, and a couple of times I have gotten lost driving home from my office."

Suddenly a chill went through me. This was not good, not good at all. I suggested foregoing the pain diary and instructed her to see a physician as soon as possible.

B did see her doctor, and unfortunately received the worst possible diagnosis: a very aggressive form of non-operable brain cancer. She passed away about five months after our visit.

Besides the tragic loss of a wonderful person, there is a deep lesson in this experience. When the pieces of the puzzle do not fit, do not force them to do so. Those pieces belong to a different puzzle. What we treat, as soft tissue therapists, is mechanical pain. Mechanical pain can be made better or worse with movement or position. The client should be able to do something that will aggravate or alleviate the discomfort. In addition, if muscles are involved, muscle length or strength is almost always affected. Local tissue tenderness may be present, yet clinically irrelevant. Most importantly, recognizing that the problem isn't muscular will facilitate seeking the appropriate provider more quickly. In B's case, probably nothing could have been done to save her. In someone else, discriminating mechanical pain may be a life-saving decision. If you haven't seen someone in your practice who presents with non-mechanical pain like B, your day is coming. Be ready.

When You Name It, You Frame It

"I cannot thank you enough for telling me that! I had assumed a totally different outcome," I exclaimed. As soon as this massage therapist shared this news about a client she had referred to me months earlier, my mind went back to the moment I first saw that client, M, in my office.

Coming around the corner of my waiting room, remember seeing M sitting in an awkward position in one of the chairs. His countenance was one of what I would best describe as resignation. It's a look I have seen many times and I always know that challenges lie ahead. Facial expressions like that are earned over long-suffering struggles. M was no different.

Watching M walk from the waiting room to my treatment room, it was obvious that he was limping. It was also obvious that his pelvis was not level (pelvic obliquity). If it is so obvious as to be seen when walking, it must be significant.

"Can you tell me what symptoms you experience? When did this start? Can you give me an idea about your activity levels?" I inquired.

"This started about three months ago. My job is sedentary as I am a dentist, but I have completed several marathons, including one earlier this year. I'm not fast, but I have completed every marathon I have entered. The pain I am experiencing now just keeps escalating every day. Now, I'm not sure I could run three blocks."

"And the pain you feel?" I asked.

"I have pain down my right leg, which was diagnosed as by the orthopedist as sciatica. It goes down here (pointing to the right bicep femoris) and to the calf and foot. The surgery they want to do is a fusion of L5 / S1, as they saw a small to moderate disc issue that may be intruding on the nerve. The MRI also revealed a spondylothesis of about 5 mm, and the orthopedist would like to stabilize that as well. I am just hesitant to do all of this because, as I shared with the orthopedist, I have never really had a day of back pain in my life. It's hard to see my back as the source of the problem when my back never hurts. But, the orthopedist was less than thrilled when I questioned his diagnosis.

To be honest, I am seeing you today for two possible outcomes. If I do need the surgery, I would at least like to be more comfortable up to that point. I know this may be an unrealistic goal, but the absolute best outcome is that you could help me avoid the surgery altogether."

At this point, I was thinking that this was pretty straightforward. I often see people with back and sciatic pain who wish to avoid surgery. Research demonstrates that if you can manage through the initial pain, the end result will likely be quite good. Just as I was thinking I knew where this session was headed, the wheels fell off the wagon.

"I also feel pain from the top of my hip to the buttocks area. That pain can often wrap around the front of the hip and go to the inside of the knee. I feel that pain just as often, perhaps more lately, than the other pain to the calf and foot."

While I did not say anything to M, this was perplexing. This pain to the front of the thigh and the medial knee is not typical in the least for an L5 distribution. What would explain this? Perhaps another spinal segment higher than L5? What were the chances of having two separate areas of lumbar problems and still no experience of back pain?

At that point, I reflected on his obliquity presentation in the waiting room and asked him to stand. There was a visible discrepancy and the right hip not only looked higher but was visibly larger. Asking him to lie supine on the table, I measured his leg length. The right was significantly longer.

"Has anyone mentioned to you the possibility that you have an anatomically short left leg" I asked.

"Funny you should ask. My wife is a physical therapist and she mentioned the same thing the other day. I have been seeing other therapists in her office, and all of them commented on my leg length."

What I could not shake was the image of his hip being not only superior, but physically larger. That led me to closely look at his face. Looking very closely, it was clear that one whole side of his face was smaller than the other.

"I have a goofy question, if you don't mind. Is your left foot the same size as your right foot?" I asked with a hint of hesitation.

M gave me a look of astonishment.

"Why, yes, my left foot is smaller than my right. How in the world..." he said as his voice trailed off.

"Do you think this is the cause of my pain?" M wondered.

"It is certainly possible, but we should at least consider other choices," I answered.

I did lightly consider other possible reasons, but I was distracted with his anatomical discrepancy. I must admit that the overwhelming emphasis of the session was related to his hemipelvis.

When I saw M a week later, his wife joined him for the appointment. She was very intrigued with my observation of his hemipelvis, which was then confirmed by her physical therapy colleagues. She had many questions about how I knew to look for this, but I was distracted by her husband's report.

"I feel like my pants don't fit as well as they did, even two weeks ago. This is crazy distortion is getting worse," he revealed.

That revelation troubled me deeply. Distortions like a hemipelvis don't get worse in such a short time. More troubling, his pain had not lessened, but was steadily and slowly increasing. It was time to rethink the whole approach.

"Is there any position that alleviates or aggravates your pain?" I asked, frustrated that I neglected to ask that question at his first appointment.

"Not really," he replied. This was not the answer I was hoping for. Pain due to soft tissue should be influenced by position or movement; that was not happening for M. Why not? What would explain his pain?

Palpating his hip more carefully, I felt tissue restriction that was unlike anything I had previously felt. There was a circular area of about 10 cm that was very firm and with clear margins. I lingered long over the area, trying to process what I was feeling. His wife noticed my focus.

"Do you feel something unusual?" she asked.

"I do," I replied. "Come feel this with me."

"What do you think that is?" she questioned. "I have never felt anything like that, but I've only been in practice for three years."

"I have been in practice for almost forty years, but I have never felt anything like this either. I must admit I am baffled as to what this means. I don't like what I feel. I think we should get this checked out."

"I've got another appointment with the orthopedist in two weeks or so. I could ask him to take a look at this," M interjected.

I had to respond in a far more direct way than I am used to doing with a client. "Please pardon me for being direct, but I think this should be checked out tomorrow and by someone other than the orthopedist. See a different doctor and focus your complaint on hip pain. Don't say anything about pain down the leg. Do whatever it takes to get them to do an MRI of your hip. Really, do it tomorrow."

I will never forget the look his wife gave me as they left the office that day. She was terrified, and her eyes showed it. I kept seeing her face for the rest of the day, knowing that if I was wrong, I needlessly caused two people much extra anguish and worry. Not a pleasant thought.

A week later, I received a text from M. He had been diagnosed with a very aggressive from of cancer in his hip and while he in shock at the diagnosis, he was enormously appreciative of the help and direction I gave him. The oncologist had very nice things to say as well, very appreciative that a massage therapist displayed such good clinical reasoning skills. These were nice affirmations, but I couldn't stop thinking about the ordeal that M was facing. His last communication with me was that he was moving to be near a major cancer center.

I thought of M from time to time after that, wondering how he was doing. I had forgotten the name of the therapist who referred him to me, so I could not ask for an update. Worse yet, internet searches for his dentistry practice turned up nothing. I assumed the worst, which brings us back to the beginning of this story. I happened to run into the referring therapist at a national conference and she thanked me for taking good care of M. She also relayed that although he may likely lose a leg, he has a good chance of living through this ordeal. I was overjoyed to hear that he was still alive.

There is a larger lesson in this saga, one that deals with the danger of naming a condition. In essence, when you name it, you frame it. What M had was pain down the leg. Sciatic pain is pain down the leg, but all pain down the leg is not sciatic pain. There are many other possible reasons. Once you name it sciatica, you also assume that the problem originates in the lumbar spine. This, of course, is why the orthopedist did an MRI of the back. Finding very little pathology did not deter him from assuming that no matter the degree of discal issues, the problem must start in the lumbar spine. He ignored M's statement about never having back pain, because that statement didn't fit the preferred model.

For every client I see, I ask myself two very important questions.

1. What makes me think that the problem is soft-tissue in origin? (My expertise can also be my blind spot, where soft tissue is the reason for every pain.)
2. What else could explain this symptom?

Had the orthopedist asked himself the second question, M might have seen an oncologist sooner. Had I asked myself (and M) the first question on session number one, I'd have referred him sooner as well.

We could all be better. It's a lesson, and a client, that I won't forget.

The 2%

"Did you have to go to school for that?"

Ever had someone ask you that question? For most of us in the massage therapy field, we heard it more than a few times over the years. Quite simply, massage therapy is much deeper than what is revealed at first glance. Yes, you can teach anyone to rub someone's back using traditional strokes in a relatively short period of time. That is not massage therapy. Sensing, responding, and deriving meaning from what is sensed is a whole different matter. If you hand me a golf club and tell me to get the golf ball in the little hole, you have now explained the entire goal of the game of golf. Executing this task is another matter. While I can stand over a golf ball, I have no idea what I am doing other than to get the ball in the hole. A professional golfer is reacting and responding to stimuli I don't even know exist. Worse yet, I cannot perceive a golfer's internal processes just by watching him. I just see someone standing over a ball. They have a world of experiences that I cannot see and therefore cannot know without some training and insight.

I often tell my clients after a session that I hope they had as much fun as I did. I am sincere in that statement. The internal pictures in my head, the reactions to their tissue, the mysteries of figuring out the correlation of their presenting symptoms with their initial narrative, the way referral patterns are individual and unique; all of these factors make the work endlessly fascinating and challenging. Yet, none of these processes are visible to the client. In the end, it is my hands touching their body. In reality, the whole experience is far deeper and richer.

Reacting and responding also implies a process that is dynamic rather than static. This is at the heart of Precision Neuromuscular Therapy. The core of PNMT is reasoning, not recipes. Recipes have their place, but they have severe limitations. In the field of soft-tissue therapy, imposing a protocol on a client is like saying "I have a fabulous answer and I hope it matches your question."

Jakob Bernoulli, in his book *Ars Conjectandi* (published posthumously in 1713), used the phrase "Ars Conjectandi sive Stochastice" ("The Art of Conjecturing or Stochastics"). Translated, this phrase is perhaps the first reference to the stochastic arts. Stochastic arts imply a certain level of randomness in the process, that there are unforeseen twists and turns in the process. A sculptor may have an idea of what he wishes to create, but an imperfection in the medium (perhaps the marble), might take the art in a new direction. An improv actor may be surprised in the way another actor responds to his prompting, but that new idea takes the skit in a new and much better direction. It is the process of unpredictability that makes the art so deeply compelling for the creator. We, as the viewers of the end product, do not see the richness and depth of the process that created it.

One of my clients, a mechanical engineer, is great friends with an orthopedic surgeon, and they often watch surgery training videos together in the doctor's basement. Viewing yet another instructional video, the engineer boldly stated to the surgeon, "I think that with my engineering background, 98% of what you do, I could do." Several seconds passed. Smiling thoughtfully, the surgeon answered. "That might be true," he said. "But it's the other 2% that matters." Point. Set. Match.

For me, the other 2% is the ability to adapt and redirect a session when things do not go as planned. If you see enough clients with soft tissue pain, you have extensive experience in things not going according to plan. These difficult cases are the ones that challenge you the most, and what challenges you, changes you. Real learning happens in the struggle and constant adaptation. That is why I so value being in the clinic every day, seeing people in pain. The twists and turns of problem solving are where the richness lives. It's the other 2% that matters.